THE HEALTH CARE SUPERVISOR

EFFECTIVE EMPLOYEE RELATIONS

Edited by
Charles R. McConnell
Vice President for Employee Affairs
The Genesee Hospital
Rochester, New York

AN ASPEN PUBLICATION®
Aspen Publishers, Inc.
Gaithersburg, Maryland
1993

ST. PHILIP'S COLLEGE LIBRARY

Library of Congress Cataloging-in-Publication Data

The health care supervisor on effective employee relations /
[edited by] Charles R. McConnell
p. cm.
Includes bibliographical references and index.
ISBN: 0-8342-0366-9
1. Health facilities—Personnel management.
2. Supervision of employees. I. McConnell, Charles R.
[DNLM: 1. Personnel Management.
2. Health Facilities—organization & administration.
WX 15 H43453 1993]
RA971.35.H425 1993
362.1'1'0683—dc20
DNLM/DLC
for Library of Congress
93-196
CIP

Copyright © 1993 by Aspen Publishers, Inc.
All rights reserved.

Aspen Publishers, Inc. grants permission for photocopying for limited personal or internal use. This consent does not extend to other kinds of copying, such as copying for general distribution, for advertising or promotional purposes, for creating new collective works, or for resale. For information, address Aspen Publishers, Inc., Permissions Department, 200 Orchard Ridge Drive, Suite 200, Gaithersburg, Maryland 20878.

Editorial Resources: Barbara Priest

Library of Congress Catalog Card Number: 93-196
ISBN: 0-8342-0366-9

Printed in Canada

1 2 3 4 5

Contents

Part I   The Supervisory Focus

Part II   The Supervisor and the Employee

among employees to what they perceive as growing organizational control over their lives and work.

Part III   Some Special Problems and Processes

Part IV Major Redirections

Preface

INTRODUCTION

The Health Care Supervisor is a cross-disciplinary journal that publishes articles of relevance to persons who manage the work of others in health care settings. This journal's readers, as well as its authors, come from a wide variety of functional, clinical, technical, and professional backgrounds. Between the covers of a single issue of *HCS,* for example, you can find articles written by a nurse, a physician, a speech pathologist, a human resource specialist, an accountant, a nursing home administrator, and an attorney. These authors, and the numerous others who write for *HCS,* write with a single purpose: To provide guidance that all health care supervisors, regardless of the occupations or specialties they supervise, can use in learning to better understand or fulfill the supervisory role.

Getting work done through other people necessitates regarding each employee as a whole person, not simply as a producer of output. The employee as a person cannot be successfully separated from the employee as a producer; to direct the latter is to deal with the former as well. In *The Health Care Supervisor on Effective Employee Relations,* we have brought together 22 articles that provide insight into a wide range of employee relations concerns.

THE SUPERVISORY FOCUS

"The Evolution of Employee Relations: A New Look at Criticism and Discipline" sets the stage for consideration of employee relations in the 1990s and beyond. In "A Management Credo", Norman Metzger reminds us that leadership by outstanding example remains the preferred way to move the work group toward common goals. Likewise, with "Human Resources Management: Keystone for Productivity", Bruce Bartels and Keith Gee reinforce the necessity to continually place people first in the process of securing output. Recognizing that the supervisor controls many of the conditions affecting motivation in the group, in "Worker Perception: The Key to Motivation", Paul Fitzgerald reveals that what the employees perceive to be so can be more important in governing their actions than what is actually so.

THE SUPERVISOR AND THE EMPLOYEE

"Employee Clout: Who's Running This Organization, Anyway?" acknowledges the necessity of changing with the times and remaining current in the present era of increasing awareness of individual rights, while "The Visible Supervisor" reminds all supervisors that it has always been and forever will be important for the supervisor to be visible and available to the staff.

In "A Supervisory Challenge: The Difficult Employee", Joan Moore points out that some employees inevitably require more supervisory attention than others, and Douglas Dorman, in "Dealing With the Angry Employee", prepares us to counter constructively when addressing employee anger. Further, in "Dealing With People Who Fail to Produce", William Umiker shows that employee problems have many different possible causes and thus many different paths toward solution.

In "Handling Manipulation and Responding to the Codependent Employee", Ruth Davidhizar addresses two significant areas of frequent concern to the supervisor, and joined by Margaret Bowen she encourages the supervisor in moving the staff forward against seemingly hopeless opposition in "When the Manager Encounters, 'We Can't Do It!'."

To close out this section, in "Managing Organizational Aversion Among Employees", Howard Smith and Neill Piland discuss how supervisors can help employees cope with some of the disadvantages of being a very small part of a very large, complex, sometimes seemingly impersonal organization.

SOME SPECIAL PROBLEMS AND PROCESSES

The "Manager as a Conflict Negotiator" by Rita Numerof introduces the supervisor's vital role in bringing solutions and compromises into an arena of problems and differences. In "Absenteeism: A Nurse Manager's Concern", Kip DeWeese reflects a valid concern of all who manage the work of others. Carol Distasio, in "How to Delegate Effectively", offers down-to-earth practical guidance for the development of a supervisor's essential delegation skills.

The "Supervisor's Role in the Discipline and Grievance Process" finds Norman Metzger sharing many years of knowledge and experience in these critical employee relations activities.

In "Team Building Techniques for the Health Care Supervisor" Jerry Norville reveals how to forge a cohesive, mutually directed work unit from a collection of individuals, and Charlotte Eliopoulos provides for the supervisor's appreciation of the value of a dedicated personnel health office in "Employee Health Services: A Mutually Beneficial Program for Facility and Staff."

MAJOR REDIRECTIONS

In "Challenging Change", Jon Tris Lahti proposes that often the best reaction to that which is new is neither resistance nor blind acceptance but rather thoughtful questioning of the elements of the change.

Carole Fink, in "The Impact of Mergers on Employees", prepares supervisors in the ways to prepare their employees for the major adjustments necessitated by mergers of health care organizations. From "Planning and Implementing a Staff Reduction" by William Weimer and Paul Cutlip, supervisors learn of their role in the unpleasant but sometimes necessary process of reducing the size of the organization.

CONCLUSION

Effective employee relations is a pursuit that lasts as long as one's employment as a manager. As long as one has direct-reporting employees there will be employee problems. Satisfactory relations with the employees in the work group is a continuing concern for the health care supervisor second to all employees' concern for patient care.

Acknowledgments

It would not have been possible to assemble this book without the active involvement of the members of the guiding boards, past and present, of *The Health Care Supervisor*. As of this writing some of these valued advisors and authors are well into their second decade of service to *HCS*.

Our sincere thanks to the following past members of the *HCS* Editorial Board, present members of the *HCS* Advisory Board, and present members of the Board of Contributing Editors.

Past Members of Editorial Board

Steven H. Appelbaum, Zeila W. Bailey, Claire D. Benjamin, Marjorie Beyers, Philip Bornstein, Leonard C. Brideau, Robert W. Broyles, Joy D. Calkin, Kenneth P. Cohen, Joseph A. Cornell, Darlene A. Dougherty, Kenneth R. Emery, Valerie Glesnes-Anderson, Lee Hand, Allen G. Herkimer, Jr., Max G. Holland, Bowen Hosford, Charles E. Housley, Loucine M. D. Huckabay, Laura L. Kalick, Janice M. Kurth, Marlene Lamnin, Joan Gratto Liebler, Ellyn Luros, Margeurite R. Mancini, Robert D. Miller, Joan F. Moore, Victor J. Morano, Harry E. Munn, Jr., Michael W. Noel, Rita E. Numerof, Samuel E. Oberman, Cheryl S. O'Hara, Jesus J. Pena, Donald J. Petersen, Tim Porter-O'Grady, George D. Pozgar, Ann Marie Rhodes, Edward P. Richards III, James C. Rose, Rachel Rotkovich, Norton M. Rubenstein, Edward D. Sanderson, William L. Scheyer, Homer H. Schmitz, Joyce L. Schweiger, Donna Richards Sheridan, Margaret D. Sovie, Eugene I. Stearns, Judy Ford Stokes, Thomas J. Tenerovicz, Lewis H. Titterton, Jr., Dennis A. Tribble, Terry Trudeau, Alex J. Vallas, Katherine W. Vestal, Judith Weilerstein, William B. Werther, Jr., Shirley Ann Wertz, Sara J. White, Norman H. Witt, and Karen Zander

Present Advisory Board

Addison C. Bennett, Bernard L. Brown, Jr., Karen H. Henry, Norman Metzger, I. Donald Snook, Jr., and Helen Yura-Petro

Present Board of Contributing Editors

Donald F. Beck, Robert Boissoneau, Jerad D. Browdy, Vicki S. Crane, Carol A. Distasio, Charlotte Eliopoulos, Howard L. Lewis, R. Scott MacStravic, Leon McKenzie, Jerry L. Norville, Stephen L. Priest, Howard L. Smith, and John L. Templin, Jr.

Our sincere appreciation as well to those who, in addition several persons mentioned above, participated in creating the articles that make up this present volume: Bruce M. Bartels, Margaret Bowen, Paul W. Cutlip, Ruth Davidhizar, Kip DeWeese, D. Douglas Dorman, Carole A. Fink, Paul E. Fitzgerald, Jr., Keith L. Gee, Jon Tris Lahti, Neill F. Piland, William Umiker, and William Weimer.

Part I
The Supervisory Focus

The evolution of employee relations: a new look at criticism and discipline

Charles R. McConnell
Vice President for Employee Affairs
The Genesee Hospital
Rochester, New York

EVER SINCE organizations were formed and first engaged employees to perform work, there have been both employee problems and problem employees. Probably no supervisor with more than a few weeks' experience has not found it necessary to criticize some aspect of employee conduct or performance. Also, most working supervisors of even modest experience have had to take disciplinary action against certain employees from time to time. Although disciplining is not likely among the more favored tasks of supervisors, most will nevertheless concede the necessity to take such action on occasion.

It is likely that criticism and discipline will always be active elements of the supervisory role. However, criticism and discipline are approached differently today than they were a number of years ago, and the coming years will likely see the way

Health Care Superv, 1986,4(2),80–88
© 1986 Aspen Publishers, Inc.

ST. PHILIP'S COLLEGE LIBRARY

in which they are approached altered still further. Criticism will of course always remain criticism, and disciplinary action will likewise remain just that; however, over the years the *why* and *how* of criticism and discipline have changed dramatically and promise to change still more in years to come.

How criticism and discipline are handled in any particular work organization has always been largely dependent on the prevailing approach to organizational management. Society's general approach to organizational management has undeniably changed over time, so the treatment of criticism and discipline has understandably changed as well.

The majority of today's work organizations appear to be in the second of three phases of employee relations. These phases may be described as:

- *authoritarianism,* dating back to the time when one person first employed another and ending—at least legally, if not altogether factually—in the early 1960s;
- *legalism*—the reliance on laws, rules, and regulations—that essentially constitutes today's approach; and
- *humanism,* the likely direction of the future, in which each employee will be genuinely regarded as a whole person and not simply as a worker.

Overlying all three phases, from the final few decades of true authoritarianism onward, is the approach to running a business organization that is broadly referred to as the *human relations school of management.*

A new look at criticism and discipline necessitates examining how criticism and discipline have fared to date in the phases in employee relations, and how they will likely fare in the years to come, as influenced by the gradual, widespread adoption of the human relations philosophy of management.

THE AUTHORITARIAN PHASE: A STARTING POINT

In organizational life it was assumed for centuries that the boss was indeed the boss, and that the boss did pretty much as the boss pleased. However, this is not to suggest that all bosses were always bad and that all employees were always mistreated.

In the past the majority of management structures were indeed autocratic. Many were even strict exploitative autocracies in which workers were deliberately and systematically exploited for the direct personal benefit of the bosses (who were usually the owners). Some management structures, however, were benevolent autocracies; as long as employees did as they were told in all matters they would be treated kindly and their basic needs would be met. The benevolent autocracy is of course the paternalistic organization, exhibiting the father-knows-best approach in employee relations that even today is still to be found in some organizations.

Whether exploitative or benevolent autocracies, however, authoritarian management structures have always operated on some common assumptions about people. The *classical theory of organizational management* long held that workers were motivated primarily by economic rewards. The organization itself was characterized by clearly defined divisions of labor and a distinct authority structure.[1]

Common assumptions and Theory X

The assumptions of the classical theory are essentially those of McGregor's well-known *Theory X*.[2] Theory X holds that unless persuaded, rewarded, controlled, and punished, people will by nature remain passive and perhaps even resistant to organizational needs. Early in the twentieth century the classical theory solidified under the widely applied label of *scientific management*, arising from the work of Frederick Taylor.[3]

As far as criticism and discipline were concerned, in the authoritarian phase of employee relations, whether the prevailing mode was referred to as classical theory or scientific management, the supervisor could do almost anything without risking meaningful reaction. In many organizations the supervisor could criticize or discipline or even discharge essentially at will. The supervisor could do as he or she pleased, and as long as this conduct was consistent with the philosophy of the organization the supervisor would never have to answer for an individual action even if such was inherently unfair.

The demise of authoritarianism

The authoritarian phase more or less officially came to an end in the early 1960s. Were one to designate the major milestone at the end of the authoritarian phase, the turning point in spelling the end of the legal toleration of widespread authoritarianism, it would probably be the Civil Rights Act of 1964. Of course the authoritarian phase of employee relations simply did not come to a complete, abrupt halt in 1964. There are carryover elements of authoritarianism that have contributed significantly to the legalistic phase of employee relations. Also, authoritarianism was not necessarily healthy and thriving right up to the moment of its legal demise. During its latter decades authoritarianism was eroded by a weakening of scientific management owing to the introduction and spread of the human relations school of management.

THE HUMAN RELATIONS APPROACH: OLD ASSUMPTIONS WEAKEN

Although Frederick Taylor stood very nearly alone in advancing scientific management, there were many contributors to the development of the human relations approach. Probably the earliest leading figure in the human relations movement was Elton Mayo, who with a team of associates guided the well-known "Hawthorne studies" at the Western Electric Company's Hawthorne Works in Chicago from 1927 to 1932.[4]

The general conclusions arising from the Hawthorne studies, now seeming to represent little more than common sense but at the time appearing to be extremely revealing, were

- The economic incentive is not the only significant or valid motivating force. Output is also influenced by an employee's relations with other workers and by personal problems experienced on and off the job.
- The worker responds not as an isolated individual but rather as a member of a work group. People working together tend to build up an informal organization that may or may not have goals similar to or parallel with the goals of the formal organization.

People working together tend to build up an informal organization that may or may not have goals similar to or parallel with the goals of the formal organization.

- Extremely refined task specialization does not necessarily make for maximum productive efficiency. What is gained through specialization can readily be lost through the effects of repetition and inflexibility.

Throughout the Hawthorne studies, as job factors were manipulated for better or worse to test the effects on employees and their output, one observation emerged repeatedly: People were often responding favorably for but one apparent reason— *someone was paying attention to them.*

Requisites to best efforts

The human relations approach to management generally holds that most people will do their best when they are treated with respect, recognized as individuals, and made to feel a meaningful part of the organization. Presently, in this sixth decade since the start of the Hawthorne studies, the human relations movement continues to flourish and expand. Human motivation relative to work is still widely studied and written about; there is even good reason to suggest that only recently has the full range of the complexity of human motivation begun to emerge.

Human-relations–oriented management techniques, such as work simplification, management by objectives, job enrichment, and quality circles, continue to emerge and proliferate. Although each such technique seems to come on the scene as a cure-all, or at least as a marvelous new management gimmick, each, after enjoying a period of fadlike popularity, settles in to become an occasionally used tool in management's bag of tricks. Although such techniques have enjoyed widely varying degrees of acceptance and success, all have something significant in common— all are aimed at improving output and enhancing organizational relationships by inspiring the active participation of the person who does the job. Also, concepts such as *quality of work life* (QWL)—demonstrated in the QWL movement—go to great lengths to acknowledge the producer as a whole person, recognizing that those who overall are the happiest and most fulfilled are also those who produce best.

Theory Y

The positive assumptions about people inherent in the human relations approach to management are generally recognizable as the basis of McGregor's *Theory Y*.[5] Theory Y holds that if people are treated as responsible contributors they will behave as responsible contributors.

From the Hawthorne experience onward, the human relations approach has steadily chipped away at the foundations of classical authoritarian management, but the human relations approach made a quantum leap forward as some major elements of the authoritarian phase of employee relations were removed by the power of legislation.

THE LEGALISTIC PHASE: A STEP FORWARD

In the previous issue of *The Health Care Supervisor* (4:1, October 1985) there appeared a discussion entitled, "Employee Clout: 'Who's Running This Organization, Anyway?'" This examination of the changing status of the individual relative to the organization pointed out that before 1964 there were essentially no major avenues of legal recourse for employees outside of their employing organizations. However, since the passage of the Civil Rights Act of 1964 and a number of other related laws, there have been an increasing number of legal avenues made available to employees who believe they have been discriminated against in any aspect of employment (hiring, promotion, transfer, layoff, etc.) and to employees who believe they have been unfairly disciplined or unjustly discharged.

Of course there were certain legal protections available for employees before 1964. There were federal and state labor laws governing hours of work and working conditions, some in effect since the 1930s and earlier (although it has been only since 1967 that health care workers have been protected by the minimum wage and overtime provisions of the federal Fair Labor Standards Act). However, it was indeed as late as the early and middle 1960s when employee protection against discriminatory and arbitrary treatment began to emerge in force. Prior to 1964 the supervisor could hire, transfer, promote, discipline, or fire for any number of inherently unfair reasons and get away with it as long as he or she did not violate the edicts of management or the policies of the organization. Now, however, the supervisor clearly cannot do so, and the policies of the organization will generally not support doing so. If an aggrieved employee is a member of a recognized minority group, or of any group for which specific laws are needed for protection of rights, the supervisor and the organization may have to deal with discrimination charges brought by any of several arms of government. Even if an aggrieved employee is not clearly a member of a recognized minority or of such a group, the supervisor could nevertheless have to deal with legal charges of unjust or unfair treatment and with lawsuits brought by individuals.

Amid the regulatory pressures of the legalistic phase of employee relations, criticism and discipline have become formalized as parts of a process that must always demonstrate that an effort has been made to correct a person's behavior and turn it toward acceptable or productive behaviors. As often as not, criticism is now the initial counseling or oral warning step in what has come to be known as *progressive discipline.*

Given the direction that applicable laws have taken regarding discharge from employment, unless it occurs for clearly provable gross misconduct as defined in the organization's work rules and supported by law, any firing is likely to be examined outside the organization with one key question in mind: Was the employee given every reasonable opportunity to correct the offending behavior?

Many of today's experienced working supervisors are aware of the rules they must follow in disciplining their workers. Many have also had cause to become aware of the organizational checks and balances that exist to ensure that the rules are followed. However, appropriate checks and balances are not always present, and even when they are present they do not always work. Overall, most supervisors seem to gravitate toward being of one of two minds: those who know the rules fairly well but see the outside employee advocacy organizations as adversaries attempting to force them to comply with rules through the threat of punishment; and those who do not know the rules, or who, if knowing the rules, ignore them, adhering (if only subconsciously) to the authoritarian philosophy of management.

What makes the present phase of employee relations legalistic is largely a matter of supervisory attitude. For example, in a continuing education session concerned with progressive disciplinary processes, after reviewing the organization's multistep process, a number of supervisors were asked: Why do you believe you need to apply this process fully to each problem employee? The supervisors' responses included:

- "We will get a complaint from (the State Division of) Human Rights if I do not."
- "I do not want to get in trouble by bringing the Equal Employment Opportunity Commission down on us."
- "I might cause us to get sued."
- "It is policy. I have to follow it."

In reality, however, the philosophical basis of progressive discipline is far removed from the implications of the foregoing reflections of legal requirements backed up with negative repercussions. The philosophical basis of progressive discipline is actually

- to afford the employee every reasonable opportunity to correct inappropriate behavior before it becomes serious enough to result in termination (and not simply to *demonstrate* to others that this opportunity has been extended);
- to attempt true corrective action (and not simply to provide *documentation* of attempts at correction); and
- to make every reasonable effort to help the employee become a productive contributor (and not simply to *remove* the unproductive employee).

The laws, rules, and regulations presently governing employee treatment are seen by many as limitations and constraints on management's ability to manage. Yet in mandating fair and equal treatment of all employees, the laws and their implementing regulations are intended to channel supervisors into working constructively in an effort to salvage each problem employee. However, instead of approaching each case by attempting to determine what can be done to make a troublesome employee more productive, many supervisors are in effect trying to determine what can be done to get rid of

It is the reasons behind the adherence to laws and regulations that make the difference between the legalistic phase and the humanistic phase of employee relations.

the substandard performer with minimal risk of adverse reaction.

Thus the legalistic phase of employee relations is a phase in which many of the right steps are being taken, but often they are taken for the wrong reasons. It is the reasons behind the adherence to laws and regulations that make the difference between the legalistic phase and the humanistic phase of employee relations. As one human resource manager expressed the problem, "I'm frequently asked something like, 'How can I legally get rid of this employee?' For years we simply clubbed employees. We still do it, but now we club them *legally*."

THE HUMANISTIC PHASE: THE SHAPE OF THE FUTURE

One will of course recognize that there are not clear-cut divisions between the phases of employee relations. Although we are more than two decades into the legalistic phase there are still pockets of authoritarianism to be found, many of them in smaller businesses not covered by prevailing laws. Similarly, there are entire organizations, as well as supervisors within organizations, that practice humanistic employee relations. The legalistic phase of today is a lengthy transition period during which habits and attitudes are changing and new management philosophies are evolving.

Major change, especially change in habits and attitudes, often occurs gradually and is usually difficult. Many of today's supervisors began their management careers during the authoritarian phase—the boss may not necessarily have always been right, but the boss was always the boss. Even many younger supervisors, those entering management long after the start of the legalistic phase, have been subject to strong authoritarian influences. These newer supervisors have had as role models managers whose attitudes and behavior reflect authoritarianism. The attitudes born of the legalistic phase—rules are rules, and like them or not we have to follow them—will likely take years to work themselves through and give way to healthier attitudes. The humanistic phase will have arrived when the supervisor no longer thinks, "I need to follow these steps because it is required of me," but rather thinks, "I need to do these things because I want to salvage this employee if at all possible."

The prevailing legalistic human relations approach has indeed solved some old problems, but it has also created a number of new problems that only a humanistic approach can solve. Consider, for example, a common problem such as chronic absenteeism.

The present legalistic approach generally requires consistency in dealing with absenteeism from one employee to another. Thus if the chronic abuser of sick time is disciplined, so also must the employee experiencing legitimate chronic illness or other personal or family problems be disciplined for excessive absenteeism. As harsh as this may sound to some, there is nevertheless a certain logic in such consistent treatment—regardless of the reasons for an employee's absence, be these reasons capricious or legitimate, the fact remains that the absent employee's work either does not get done or must be accomplished at additional expense and inconvenience. In the present legalistic phase of employee relations the employee who is chronically absent from work is likely to be separated from employment regardless of the reasons behind the poor attendance record.

The humanistic phase of employee relations will likely see widespread adoption of *employee assistance programs* and other techniques to deal with the problems presented by the whole person. Such programs are provided to troubled employees confidentially and often with full or at least partial insurance coverage; the programs make available counseling and treatment as necessary for

- chronic illness;
- substance abuse (drugs and alcohol);
- marriage and family conflict;

- mental illness or emotional problems; and
- financial and legal problems.

Overall the goals of employee assistance programs and other such efforts are to retain experienced employees who might otherwise be lost and to help employees who have problems to help themselves before they become unemployable. In short, the humanistic phase of employee relations will recognize each employee as a whole person and will encourage every reasonable, honest effort to truly correct our employee problems rather than simply firing our problem employees.

•   •   •

There will always be the need for disciplinary processes in our work organizations. Some people occasionally, and a few people even regularly, break the rules of the organization, and disciplinary action commonly results when someone violates the organization's work rules. Prevention is one of the keys to reducing disciplinary action, and much disciplinary action can be prevented through attention to the organization's work rules. Generally, work rules should be

- as few, as simple, and as clear as possible;

- communicated clearly to employees and reinforced with them periodically;
- perceived by employees as reasonable, equitable, and fair; and
- enforced promptly, justly, humanely, and consistently.

Unfortunately many people equate discipline with punishment when such is not always the case. The word discipline comes from disciple, one who learns or follows. Thus the appropriate emphasis to place on the word discipline is to teach—in the context of a work organization, to teach the job, the rules, and the expectations of the organization. The concept of discipline as a teaching process provides considerable challenge for the supervisor. The challenge may seem great indeed, but the potential rewards are great. There is little satisfaction to be gained from simply getting rid of a substandard performer. This may be so at least in part because the firing of an employee—even an employee who has caused problem after problem and has continually done substandard work—suggests some measure of failure on the part of the supervisor. However, there is immense satisfaction to be gained from helping the occasional substandard performer become a truly productive member of the work group.

REFERENCES

1. Etzioni, A. *Modern Organizations.* Englewood Cliffs, N.J.: Prentice Hall, 1964, p. 20.
2. McGregor, D.M. "The Human Side of Enterprise." *Management Review* 46, no. 11 (1957): 22–28, 88–92.
3. Taylor, F.W. *Scientific Management.* New York: Harper, 1911.
4. Etzioni, *Modern Organizations*, 32.
5. McGregor, "The Human Side of Enterprise."

A management credo

Norman Metzger
Edmond A. Guggenheim Professor
Department of Health Care
    Management
Mount Sinai School of Medicine
Vice President for Labor Relations
Department of Labor Relations
The Mount Sinai Medical Center
New York, New York
President
American Society for Hospital
    Personnel Administration
Chicago, Illinois

IN THE BEST SELLER *In Search of Excellence* the authors share with us a marvelously revealing anecdote about the president of an organization being confronted by a scientist working for him, who has discovered a breakthrough theory; the president immediately rummages through his desk and comes up with an item, saying "Here." It is a banana—the only reward he could immediately put his hands on. If your reaction is "how bizarre" you have missed the point. It was a genuine display of recognition and appreciation. Rewarding excellent work will likely result in a repetition of that above-average performance. Any *immediate* reward is better than delayed recognition.

APPRECIATION: THE MISSING LINK

When was the last time your boss told you you were doing a good job?

Health Care Superv, 1986,4(4),29–38
© 1986 Aspen Publishers, Inc.

When was the last time you did something well, and it was immediately recognized? You probably had such a feeling of elation that it lasted not only through the day but for a protracted period of time. Through the last several decades, researchers have identified "full appreciation of work done" as number one on the list of employee needs. The reason is obvious. It is the missing link. We pay too little attention to workers' needs for recognition and appreciation. There is an old Oriental adage that "If you wish your merit to be known, acknowledge that of other people." Whether you do it with a banana or any other tangible expression of appreciation, it is essential that you acknowledge, to your employees, and in public, their accomplishments; this satisfies the key need for recognition and for feeling important. It helps them believe that they are accepted and approved by the institution and by you.

COMMUNICATION IMPROVES PRODUCTIVITY

The key to improving productivity is communicating to employees what is expected of them on the job and day to day, and whether they are measuring up to those expectations. One expert observer lists some of the more important points in the critical management process of performance evaluation:[1]

- Work performance is improved appreciably when employees know what results are expected; when they know the methods by which they will be measured; and when they know from you the priorities that have been established.
- Work performance is improved appreciably when employees believe that it is possible to influence the expected results. Too often, employees have the cynical view that no matter what they do it will not have an effect on the outcome—on the quality of service.
- The communication of results that were effected by the employee must be clear and specific.
- The communication of results (outcomes) must be immediate.

The successful supervisor is able to communicate to employees who have performed below standard, and is interested enough to commend those who have demonstrated above-standard performance. To be a supervisor includes the difficult task of informing people how they are doing. It is you, the manager, who is responsible for the performance of others. Therefore, you must periodically communicate the results of such performance. You do this best within an atmosphere or climate of approval. Here are four suggestions for improving your supervisory results:

1. Develop performance standards. You do not do a service to either the employee or the institution by setting low standards.
2. Use those standards to measure the employees' performance.

3. Take note of and display appreciation for above-par performance.
4. Let the below-par performers know that you are aware of their performance and expect it to change.

It matters not at which level a man or woman is in an organization; that individual wants to know where he or she has been, where he or she is now, and where he or she is going. Positive reinforcement tells a subordinate that he or she is on the right track. When you reinforce acceptable or exceptional behavior by verbal recognition, you will serve to extend such behavior and produce more acceptable or exceptional behavior.

PLANNING FOR PROGRESS

Supervisors must develop a new perception of communicating performance results. What is needed is a tool for planning for progress.

It is, indeed, a truism that most employees, if communicated to properly and provided necessary assistance, will improve their performance. It is the rule, rather than the exception, that employees can agree with their immediate supervisor on the aims and goals of the department and, in the larger picture, those of the institution. It is the supervisor's responsibility to be an inspiration for improvement, and to do this he or she must develop the plan for individual workers to become more efficient.

We tend to rediscover the wheel when studying how to change employee attitudes and improve productivity. Over the years, study after study directs our attention to the need to touch employees. This means getting out from behind your desk—from behind the paperwork—getting your nose out of the budget reports—and getting back to where it matters: into face-to-face contact with the employees.

The old reward system—dollars—although still listed as a significant need by employees, will not suffice as an incentive to productivity. Values of workers have changed as radically as the workers themselves. We must pay attention to building up trust. Employees just do not trust us. They tend to be cynical about rewards based on contribution. A most disturbing study indicated that workers believe that those who work hardest end up on the short end of the stick.[2] We have to turn around such negative feelings, such lack of trust. We cannot do this by analyzing everything. We cannot do this by concentrating solely on policies, organizational structures, job descriptions, or rules and regulations. Yes, all of these must be present, but we as the leaders must help people reach their full potential. We must have a sense of caring—of appreciation. Too many workers are alienated on the job. Alienation is a destructive result of paying too little attention to the supervisor–subordinate relationship, and paying too much attention to negative reinforcers such as discipline. Alienation results from employees finding no meaning in their work, finding no satisfaction from their toils, and finding no love on the job.

Your employees must know that you care. If they know that you care about them then they will care about you and about their work. There is a strong case to be made for the employee-centered supervisor, the one who is less interested in control than in results. The most productive managers attempt to organize and bring together the abundance of human competence usually found in the work arena. Who are these employee-centered supervisors? What do they do? Why are they better than others?

- They communicate more. They do not protect information from employees, but rather protect employees with information.
- They are wonderfully attuned listeners. They are able to respond positively to "silly" questions. They listen to suggestions and complaints with an attitude of fair consideration and a willingness to take appropriate actions.
- They are askers rather than tellers. They know that most human beings are looking for meaning in their work and find it when their work is appreciated.

If you treat people as individuals who, like you, need to have their dignity preserved in even the most trying situations; if you constantly impress them with your concern for their welfare by simply asking them "why" something has happened; if you let them know when they have done something good, as well as when they have done something bad; if you let them speak up, then you will not only feel good about yourself but you will have made them feel good about themselves and about you.

Half the process of communication is listening. That means sitting up and listening; it does not mean sitting back and listening. Most of us talk too much. We spend too much time explaining our positions at the expense of understanding where the other person stands. Judicious silence is the hallmark of a good communicator; when you are listening, listen for *feelings*. Pay attention to the way the other individual says things, as well as to what he or she is saying. Remember, there is no communication—that is, no effective communication—when it is going only one way. Communication is a joint effort. Sound listening habits are contagious. The better a listener the supervisor is, the better listening skills she or he will inspire.

INTRODUCING CHANGE

As a supervisor, one of your most difficult responsibilities is to introduce change. The lessons learned from the many studies conducted on productivity and relating to change is that employees who participate in the shaping of change are more likely to be receptive to the change and, therefore, are overwhelmingly more productive than those who are on the re-

> *The combination of communication, participation, and appreciation is the hallmark of successful supervision.*

ceiving end of legislated change. If the people who work for you believe that you listen to their suggestions, that you encourage and value their ideas, they are more likely to express their feelings and to make suggestions. The combination of communication, participation, and appreciation is the hallmark of successful supervision. We must accept the fact that tasks that are performed through cooperation rather than competition are more efficiently accomplished with workers exhibiting a much higher degree of motivation and morale. Most employees want to be part of a purposeful group. They want to believe that they count. They want to feel that they have a chance to satisfy their needs, to realize their aspirations. The term "feel" is used intentionally because perceptions are very important. Motivation has been described as a function of worker perceptions, of the validity and attainability of various outcomes.

BECOMING AN EFFECTIVE SUPERVISOR

At the very top of the list of effective supervisory practices is a positive relationship between the supervisor and his or her subordinates. In order to reach the top of the scale, supervisors must display a willingness to move from an authority-obedience style of supervision to an involvement-participation-commitment style. Old approaches are not working. Worker alienation is pervasive. It is reflected in high absenteeism rates, cynical attitudes of subordinates, and the feeling that there is no chance for fulfillment in work. It is your job to help people reach their full potential. It is not enough to say that people are our most important asset. You must display that truth in actions. You do this by sharing knowledge, sharing decision making, sharing credit, and sharing, and sharing, and sharing. It is telling people that you recognize when they do something right—that you appreciate their contributions. Were we asked to list the most important leadership traits—those that would ensure success—the following would likely come to mind:

1. willingness to share power;
2. respect for the dignity of others;
3. primary concern for the human aspect in management;
4. concern and attention to the development of subordinates;
5. desire to reward the above-average contributor;
6. ability to let those who do not meet standards know that fact, and to let them know how to improve; and
7. possession of a belief in basic values, human dignity, human fallibility, and human needs.

BECOMING AN EFFECTIVE ORGANIZATION

The profile of a successful organization, led by managers who view workers not as instruments and factors of production, but as indispensable resources capable of being motivated and productive under certain working conditions, includes

- emphasis on organizational informality and fluid, flexible lines of communication and reporting relationships;
- the sharing of "managerial prerogatives" with line supervisors and workers on a systematic, institutionalized basis;
- a managerial ethos that insists on the constant recognition of the importance of the institution's employees; and
- antiauthoritarian employee relations structures that encourage innovativeness and decentralized initiative at the line level.

Crisis of management

The crisis of work in America is a crisis of management in America. Agonizing over the purported loss of the "work ethic" cannot obscure the real nature of this crisis; we just have not been sharing responsibility, recognition, and rewards with our employees. The institutions that have escaped this crisis display a sense of caring, managements that listen, and supervisors who direct—through their daily dealings with their employees—their attention to building up trust and commitment. People car-

ing permeates such organizations. It is strange that it took a best seller to point out that the individual human being still counts, and that building up an organization that takes note of the key role played by the individual is the job of the entire management team. This is not an easy task within the complex hospital management structures found in this country, but once we realize that alienation is greater in situations where the employees are not allowed to participate in decision making, and that frustrations grow from inflexible organizational structures, we can concentrate on ethics and make changes.

Franklin Roosevelt once said that new ideas cannot be administered successfully by men with old ideas. We must reject old ideas and old strictures when they prove to be invalid. Bruno Bettelheim, in his book *On the Uses of Enchantment*, states: "If we hope to live not just from moment-to-moment but in true consciousness of our existence, then our greatest need and most difficult achievement is to find meaning in our lives."[3] To find meaning in our lives we must find meaning in our work. The supervisor is the facilitator along that road.

The failure of authoritarian leadership

There is a belief, disturbingly widespread, that the management style suggested here, which makes the supervisor a collaborative manager rather than a control-centered manager, is too soft—too concerned with human relations. Several years ago an article appeared in one of the prominent health care magazines that talked about benevolent, laid-back administrators being obsolete. It championed the authoritarian leader. Authoritarian leadership has failed and will continue to fail. Most of these failures can manage to temporarily make gains, but they destroy the very heart of the organization as they move through it.

The heirs of Taylorism, who dominated administration both in health care and industry, have produced inefficiencies, the list of which would be too lengthy to set down in these few pages. The legitimacy of management's unshared hegemony over the work process and work place is for these scientific managers (they like to think of themselves as scientific, but one may question that description) a *sine qua non* and the manner of its exercise makes almost impossible the motivation of the work force. These authoritarian leaders have an almost obsessive bias toward measurement and quantitative analysis. They come with an exaggerated emphasis on planning, and insist on deification of policy and procedure manuals as a substitute for genuine employee-oriented, goal-directed management. These "squashers of dissent" are blame throwers. They overlook their own mistakes.

The success of the collaborative manager

The facts are clear: Supervisors and administrators who display a sense of caring, who have refined their listening antennae and who are trust-builders, build successful organizations. The authoritarian leader breeds alienation. What heightens self-respect increases efficiency, and it is the major role of supervisors to heighten self-respect. Bullies win the day, but there is always another day. The collaborative manager can be forceful. If an employee strays from the accepted institutional behavior, the collaborative manager must be firm. There is no substitute for genuine agreement on the need to do things the right way. The challenge for supervisors is to find the handle on employee cooperation.

You have got to earn cooperative and positive behavior from employees. You do this by setting the right example; by displaying a caring attitude; and by being firm, consistent, and fair. You do this by knowing each one of your employees; knowing their personalities, interests, needs, and concerns. They must believe you care; that you take time in dealing with them as individuals. Employees still list near the top of their needs "help from my supervisor on personal problems." The reason this is high on the list is that most supervisors have been remiss in responding to that need. An unfulfilled need acts as motivator, and, in such cases, a negative motivator. In looking at organizational patterns throughout the health care system one may be led to realize that respect and care are primary ingredients of successful institutions. Those institutions that fit this description inculcate a spirit within their supervisors that has as its basis the following prescription: Get to know the people who work for you; get to know them better than you know them now; get them to believe that you care about them as human beings; set the right role model for them.

●　●　●

A productive work force does not result from rules, policies, plans, and budgets, but rather from a set of values that incorporates the respect of people and their contributions to organizational success. If you are a non-threatening and supportive leader, you will create an attractive work environment and develop a sense of commitment in your subordinates that will have a direct result on the productivity of your department. What follows is a credo for successful supervisors:

- I shall treat my subordinates as adults. I shall appropriately acknowledge the good works of my subordinates. I shall encourage and recognize excellence.
- I shall share decision making with my subordinates to the fullest extent possible.
- I shall listen to dissenters; I shall encourage diversity; I shall change my views when facts are presented that differ from those that I had understood.
- I shall not pass the buck.
- I shall, as much as possible,

reach out and touch my employees so that they understand that I care.
- I shall never scapegoat; it is a destructive practice that has negative ramifications.
- I shall find the fruit of choice in recognizing contributions; some will get a banana, some will get a tangerine, and others a nod of appreciation.

Treating workers fairly, enunciating and practicing values that recognize the need, worth, and fears of employees, is not sentimental double talk and need not be opposed nor be detrimental to the productivity and financial validity of an organization. On the contrary, it is an essential partner to scientific management. Our management credo advances the terribly simple notion that workers performing work over which they exercise no control, producing results that are not recognized, and feeling that they are not part of the organization quickly exhibit the classical manifestations of alienation: high absenteeism, low productivity, sullenness, and hostility. The classic response is that they lack discipline and respect for authority, and that they are lazy. Not so! That is a restricted focus on effects rather than an attempt to understand causes and, therefore, to consider alternate management styles. With the advent of large health care institutions and complex employee relations problems, the modern supervisor, although ennobled by techniques and methods far superior to his or her predecessor, has paid a high price for "overspecialization" and for "bottom-line management."

We are pressed to get things done at the sacrifice of achieving understanding. To the extent that supervisors develop and refine the art of communicating, they will be effective managers. To the extent that supervisors understand why employees are more cynical than ever before and are less likely to be trustful of management's intentions, they will be the developers of more productive work teams.

Supervisors are dealing with a complex new breed of employees who are far more assertive, far more knowledgeable about their rights, and far more certain about what they will and will not do.

Supervisors are dealing with a complex new breed of employees who are far more assertive, far more knowledgeable about their rights, and far more certain about what they will and will not do. These workers accept less, trust less, and want more. We cannot deal with them just by pounding our chests and ordering them to do things. We must treat them as equals, thereby becoming their equal. The art of supervision is being reshaped. Old myths are being discarded. The key element in leadership is a genuine interest in people. Although leadership does depend upon a specific situation, those leaders who express a sincere interest in the people who work for them and balance it with an interest in the work itself are the most effective. If you are to do your job properly, gain the respect and admiration of your subordinates, and obtain recognition or rewards from your superiors, then you must see beyond the day-to-day details of the job and develop your ability to understand the motivations of your subordinates; learn how to speak their language; master techniques of introducing change in the face of resistance; and control subjective evaluation and determination and replace such subjectivity with dependence on facts and logic, maintaining a keen appreciation of the other person's views and needs. You must endeavor to obtain participation of all your workers. You must build trust.

Active commitment of employees is obtained and springs from a relationship of trust. Supervisors who listen to, respect, and reward employees' contributions build up such an atmosphere of trust. They use positive reinforcement; they delegate more than other supervisors; they communicate more than other supervisors; they are not preoccupied with their own job security and their own needs; they encourage diversification; and they realize that when the worker speaks, attention must be paid.

REFERENCES

1. Kessler, T.W. "Management by Objectives." In *Handbook of Health Care Human Resources Management*, edited by Norman Metzger, 184–186. Rockville, Md.: Aspen Systems, 1981.
2. Yankelovich, D. Presentation to the National Conference on Human Resources, Dallas, Texas, October 25, 1978.
3. Bettelheim, B. *On the Uses of Enchantment.* New York: Random House, 1977, p. 48.

Human resources management: keystone for productivity

Bruce M. Bartels
Vice President for Operations
Medical Center Hospital of
  Vermont

Keith L. Gee
Employee Relations Specialist
Medical Center Hospital of
  Vermont
Burlington, Vermont

THE RELATIONSHIP between institutional productivity efforts and employee behavior often takes a back seat in the development of productivity improvement programs. A more common action is to use traditional management engineering techniques as the sole or primary approach. This article will explore the thinking behind a multifaceted productivity improvement effort that encompasses the quantitative disciplines required in any such undertaking and the less tangible human components.

Many improvement efforts, while initially successful, fail to bring about lasting productivity or quality improvements.[1] There have been costly negative results in some cases, including deterioration of quality and productivity as well as heightened labor strife.

A critical determinant of the success or failure of an effort to improve

Health Care Superv, 1987, 5(2), 47–53
© 1987 Aspen Publishers, Inc.

productivity is the breadth of purpose that management communicates for the effort.[2] The more successful organizations view their primary objectives as building a competitive, productive organization.[3] The unsuccessful organization focuses more narrowly on fine tuning existing activities, often at the cost of overlooking opportunities to correct inherent weaknesses and limitations in mission, product lines, strategies, cultures, structures, human resources, and technologies.

The question thus presented is: How do we include the concepts necessary to addressing lasting improvement in a productivity enhancement effort? Research would indicate that to successfully cope with increasingly hostile environments organizations should adopt a total systems improvement approach.[4] There are five key tasks that need to be accomplished in order to build the understanding, commitment, capabilities, and methodology necessary for improvement activities to succeed. These tasks are:

1. developing a common perspective on productivity;
2. developing a culture supportive of productivity improvement efforts;
3. maximizing human resources;
4. developing organization capabilities; and
5. continually searching for improvement.

While the foregoing tasks are listed serially, only the initial task need take place in the designated order.

Once a common perspective is achieved, the remaining items can be undertaken concurrently; they are in fact never fully completed, as they are ongoing activities in a thriving organization. The remainder of this article will examine these tasks and suggest a framework for productivity enhancement based upon them.

DEVELOPING A COMMON PERSPECTIVE ON PRODUCTIVITY

There are many different interpretations of the meaning and utilization of productivity. The varying perspectives that individuals have of productivity and the implications that they see may handicap an effort at enhancement. Clarity and consensus regarding terminology, purpose, and methodology need to be achieved.

An important element in developing a common perspective beyond that of mere definition is exposure to the reasoning behind the renewed emphasis on productivity. Among the forces now so familiar to us are:

- pressures from payers and consumers to provide the same or better quality service at equal or lower cost;
- prospective payment;
- market and price competition;
- availability of capital financing; and
- inflationary pressure on wages, benefits, supplies, utilities, and equipment.

A major factor in dealing with each of the foregoing issues is productivity improvement. Communication to hospital staff members of the positive, progressive elements of productivity improvement is critical. Leaving the impression that productivity is synonymous with austerity, loss of job security, sacrifices, or lower quality is unlikely to result in enthusiasm.

DEVELOPING A CULTURE SUPPORTIVE OF PRODUCTIVITY IMPROVEMENT

Much is being written these days about organizational culture.[5] It appears to be an essential ingredient for long-term success and is often the distinguishing characteristic between success and failure. A culture is a shared set of beliefs and behaviors. How can management set out to define and make productivity improvement a part of its culture and convince others to share in this undertaking?

There are three major steps in building a culture supportive of productivity improvement. The initial action is to define when necessary and communicate the institutional mission, values, and objectives, and to explain the role of productivity improvement in the accomplishment of these. The intent is to develop a sense of purpose behind the productivity improvement effort. Many repeated acts achieve this. Among them are periodic presentation and discussion of corporate productivity objectives in settings available to all employees; articles in internal pub-

lications; incorporation of these concepts in the annual planning cycle; and identification of this notion in performance evaluations. The awareness that is created by these actions must then be translated into commitment. Commitment is the most elusive step in developing this facet of a culture, but once it occurs individuals can collectively pursue the objective.

There are no certain ways to achieve commitment. However, commitment should spring from a common perspective of individual and organizational well-being. When there is a high degree of congruence with regard to the presence and form of threats and opportunities it is most likely that commitment will be achieved.

One mechanism for communicating that productivity improvement is a standard expectation of every staff member's job is its incorporation as an element of job performance.

One mechanism for communicating that productivity improvement is a standard expectation of every staff member's job is its incorporation as an element of job performance. A vehicle that serves this purpose is a process called performance contracting.[6]

Performance contracting is a modification of management by objectives

(MBO). It uses as a communication vehicle a set of mutually agreed upon objectives directed toward obtaining results in specific areas. The performance agreement has an impact far beyond its use as an evaluation or appraisal tool. The key areas identified for results are those that senior management selects as critical to the organization's interests for the coming year. This process has a cascading communications impact. As senior management selects key result areas, divisional and departmental managers identify objectives that represent the desired results. Discussion and negotiation between managers, which must occur to complete a performance contract, reinforce institutional direction and priority.

The requirement for identification of individual actions supporting the direction established in performance contracting also permits "buying in" to occur. A manager takes an active role in creating and defining the tasks that will constitute achievement. A sensitivity to individual autonomy and participation is thus expressed through the contract.

Once a theme is developed and shared it may be made part of the organization's culture, but it must be sustained through recycling and reinforcement. This can be done by encouraging each department to define standards for productivity, promote employee involvement in improvement opportunities, increase employee recognition for achievement, and integrate standards of productivity in individual appraisals.

MAXIMIZING HUMAN RESOURCES

Attaining improvements in productivity and quality hinges on human behavior. Recognizing that each member of a hospital staff represents a potential to be tapped is central to identifying opportunities for improvement. There are several components to addressing the human aspect of this process. One is to develop and support a positive employee relations climate. Many interrelated actions are required to build these positive relations, and they all require attention to communication.

An organization's management should express its commitment to optimizing human resources in its corporate objectives and priorities. Management evaluation schemes should focus on employee relations. Additionally, policies, procedures, and practices should be reviewed with consideration for the extent to which they support a positive climate.

As basic as the foregoing is the requirement to provide managers and supervisors with tools to assist them in establishing, monitoring, and assessing a positive climate. Instruction in the creation of this environment should be undertaken. A human resources department should have the capacity to develop educational programs providing managers with training, consulting, and coaching on employee relations matters. Incentives to emphasize a positive climate can be built into performance evaluations.

Issues of job security will inevitably arise as change is suggested and greater productivity is pursued.[7] Addressing these concerns as an initial element of the process can be of benefit to the organization as well as to the individual. An employee who perceives his or her job as secure is more likely to be productive and less likely to seek security through other employment. Issues that might result from stress, such as health or family problems, may also be minimized.

Job security, it should be noted, is not intended to mean an absolute guarantee of employment. It does, however, mean that the employer must be concerned about the welfare of the employees and must strive to project that concern. Once again, communication is key. A clear understanding of the employer's long-range plans regarding labor planning and an explanation of the environment generating these plans should be conveyed to all employees.

The organization's policies and practices dealing with work force reductions should be sensitive to employee concerns and should be known and available to all. When specific actions causing change occur, explanations of such events should be provided through in-house publications and other appropriate media. Such action will decrease the extent of incorrect information that is spread by word of mouth.

As higher levels of performance are sought through enhancements in productivity, recognition and reward for performance should become part of an organization's culture.[8] Financial and other incentives for improvement, recognition through an award system, and performance-based pay systems each have a place in developing the shared value of greater productivity. It goes almost without saying that promotion of the involvement of individual employees is a significant requirement in seeking to improve an organization's productivity.

The following should be considered when determining how to promote involvement:

- explanatory seminars on approaches used in other organizations;
- a forum giving individual managers the opportunity to demonstrate methods they have used effectively;
- training sessions in problem-solving skills for employee groups; and
- the requirement that each department select an involvement approach appropriate to its unique needs.

DEVELOPING ORGANIZATIONAL CAPABILITIES

A number of supportive capabilities must be present to sustain an ongoing productivity improvement effort. The first such required capability is the expertise to establish a productivity measurement system.[9] If productivity is to be objectively evaluated and improved, indicators for each area of activity need to be developed. This information is required to meet a number of needs. Indicators that are simple, easy to explain, and quickly calculated will help in monitoring and controlling performance. Comparative indicators that measure how an area compares with industrywide standards provide useful information as well as a competitive objective. As these indicators are developed, a method for producing relevant management reports on a periodic basis should be established as well.

As productivity can be a complex topic involving many disciplines, establishing a technical support group should be considered.

As productivity can be a complex topic involving many disciplines, establishing a technical support group should be considered.[10] This group would be available to guide and consult on various efforts taking place throughout the organization.

Representatives from several areas should be involved in the technical support group—at least membership from management engineering, quality control, personnel, data processing, and finance. Such a group can identify and catalogue institution-wide activity, provide information and expertise not generally available, and develop consistency and continuity for diverse endeavors.

Assessment tools may be as valuable as any single aid in determining where to begin.[11] Everyone becomes conditioned to their environment over time, and opportunities for change may become less visible. Assessment tools provide a structured approach to review existing systems, policies, practices, and procedures. Such tools include:

- employee relations reports;
- opinion surveys;
- internal audits;
- work simplification, work sampling, and downtime studies;
- work flow and space–relationship analyses; and
- purchasing audits and studies.

Another essential support activity is the development of a resource library.[12] This collection may be overseen by the technical support group. It should serve as a repository for information from all disciplines bearing on the topic of productivity. An organized approach for making this information available should be developed for the purpose of keeping abreast of recent developments as well as maintaining productivity efforts in a highly visible fashion.

THE ONGOING SEARCH FOR IMPROVEMENT

The final task is to continue pursuing the creation of a corporate culture having productivity as one of its primary values. Underlying this value is the assumption that anything and everything—product, cost, process, attitude, and interactions—can be improved. The integration of productivity and quality to produce greater value should be viewed as an overriding objective. It is this result that generates the rewards for initially undertaking productivity enhancement efforts.

Improvement efforts are aimed at all levels of the organization. The individual employee must be brought into the process. This may occur through various management strategies such as pay for performance, management by objectives, or quality circles. Individual actions and ideas need to be harnessed to work group, departmental, or divisional objectives. This permits capture and transmission of important innovations that benefit the activities of the group.

Integrating and supporting functions should occur at the corporate level so that achievement is recognized and enlarged upon. Supporting resources can be used to augment individual or small-group efforts and may be most effectively provided by a staff available to many people.

The new organizational culture is generated by a multidisciplinary approach aimed at various levels of the organization and arrayed in such a way as to develop a cyclic and reinforcing process. The support of individual and group efforts in pursuit of productivity that addresses the needs and experiences of the people involved will create the highest probability of success. The recognition and support of the human resources that drive productivity serve the best interests of any organization; only through behavioral change will lasting improvement be achieved.

REFERENCES

1. Goodman, P.S. "Why Productivity Programs Fail: Reasons and Solutions." *National Productivity Review* 1 (Autumn 1982): 369–80.
2. Metz, E.J. "Managing Change: Implementing Productivity and Quality Improvements." *National Productivity Review* 3 (Summer 1984) 303–13.
3. Moss, S. "A Systems Approach to Productivity." *National Productivity Review* 3 (Summer 1984) 270–79.
4. Ibid., 271.
5. Deal, T.E., and Kennedy, A.A. *Corporate Cultures*. Reading, Mass.: Addison-Wesley, 1982.
6. McDonald, C.R. *MBO Can Work! How to Manage By Contract*. New York: McGraw–Hill, 1982.
7. Mooney, M. "Organizing for Productivity Management." *National Productivity Review* 1 (Spring 1982): 141–50.
8. Shetty, Y.K. "Key Elements of Productivity Improvement Programs." *Business Horizons* 25 (March–April 1982): 15–22.
9. Kendrick, J.W. *Improving Company Productivity*. Baltimore, Md.: Johns Hopkins University Press, 1984, p. 118.
10. Bureau of Business Practice. "Centering the Productivity/Quality Effort." *Productivity Improvement Bulletin*, no. 407, January 10, 1984, 1–3.
11. Mooney, "Organizing for Productivity Management," 148.
12. Ibid.,146.

Worker perceptions: the key to motivation

Paul E. Fitzgerald, Jr.
Assistant Professor
Graduate Program in
  Health Services Administration
University of Arkansas at Little
  Rock
Little Rock, Arkansas

THE NEED FOR MOTIVATION

Why should supervisors want to motivate employees? Management literature points out many specific benefits of well-motivated employees, including increased productivity, decreased turnover, decreased absenteeism and other advantages, but the most important benefit is simply that well-motivated employees make the work environment a better place in which to function. In such an environment people are working toward goals that are important to them, and this vested interest makes the work more satisfying.

There have been some profound changes in motivational techniques and theories in the past decade. Workers themselves have changed because of numerous factors in the work environment and in society. As a result of many changes, managers and supervisors must now respond to

Health Care Superv, 1984,3(1),13–18
© 1984 Aspen Publishers, Inc.

workers and their needs differently than in the past. The days of the prevailing Protestant work ethic are gone. Work is rarely done for work's sake, and supervisors must respond to this change. Workers cannot be expected to motivate themselves or to bring the right attitudes to work, but one must instead assume that it is the supervisor's responsibility to provide the means for motivation. There is an increasing amount of pressure on the supervisor to coach, counsel and motivate workers. This pressure stems from the ever-increasing technical complexity of jobs in the health care system, changes in society as a whole and, of course, the changes in individuals. The question must now be: How can the supervisor, as part of the management team, carry out this extremely difficult and increasingly complicated task?

ALTERNATIVE APPROACHES

Before attempting to motivate workers, supervisors need to understand them and to examine the various means that cause motivation to occur. The process of motivating can be accomplished in one of three ways: (1) through intuition and experience, (2) by using scientific and quantitative methods and (3) a combination of 1 and 2.

Method 1, intuition and experience, means that one relies exclusively on feelings based on day-to-day interactions and then makes determinations about what will motivate workers. There is never direct questioning of any kind. No quantitative tools are used, and the process remains subjective.

The second method, scientific and quantitative methods, is preached about in classrooms everywhere. This approach features decisions based on objective, data-based information and tools. The tools are objective but can often be found to ignore hidden factors such as politics, general knowledge of the environment or other nonquantifiable concepts.

The third method, combining intuition and experience with an objective, scientific approach, is the preferred method. The data should be examined first and then a decision made based on how intuition or experience tempers the data. The scientific methods could include attitude surveys or any number of devices or formats. The key is to use an objective, standardized tool, which can then be examined realistically, thus providing the experiential, subjective element. This course of action should be most likely to tell supervisors what is necessary to motivate their workers.

It is vital to remember that individual workers and groups of workers differ from each other. A program, a supervisor or a policy can be as specific as possible in meeting individual needs, but an across-the-board philosophy that treats everyone the same will fail because individuals are different, seek different rewards, have different environmental needs and want various types of recognition. This situation becomes extremely complex in a health care institution because of the numerous job classifications and professions and the varied backgrounds of individual workers. A manageable and widely applied method of differentiating workers in health care institutions appears to be by job classification, i.e., RN, LPN, various types of allied health professions, housekeeper, dietary, maintenance and so on.

Levine[1] and Fitzgerald[2] found that there is no single motivator that pushes each worker; rather, a combination of motivators is generally necessary for the optimum effect, and that combination varies by job classification as well as by shift, age, sex, race and individual preference. The determination of motivational factors is extremely difficult, and the nature of the health care institution complicates the process further still.

Administrators cannot expect supervisors to motivate workers without giving some training in how to perform this function. McCreight spelled out the complexity of the supervisor's role in the motivational process by specifying five crucial roles. The supervisor must serve as: (1) goal setter, (2) trainer, (3) mentor, (4) evaluator and (5) decision maker.[3]

Levine also emphasized that supervisory skills in motivation must match desired outcomes.[4] Therefore, supervisors cannot be expected to carry out this vital and complex function of motivation without training. Unfortunately, management often leaves the unprepared supervisor to learn by doing, which is an inappro-

priate expectation that can have enormous impact on the individuals involved and cause substantial cost to the organization and its patients. Supervisors must be trained to be effective in their expected role as motivators.

WORKER PERCEPTIONS

The key in determining workers' needs and developing the appropriate motivational programs or processes is the workers' own perceptions of their needs. Remember that intuition and experience can be important in developing ideas, but policy must be developed from data that are produced by the target population. Certainly supervisors can be more confident of an attitude or a feeling if employees tell them how they feel. Of course people are not always truthful, particularly when they feel their job security may be threatened, but reliable and valid instruments produce better information for decision making than guesswork or intuition produces.

Consider a situation in which employees are offered a yearly cash bonus for perfect attendance, but supervisors find that absenteeism rates do not change. This might be so because management has never defined specifically what would motivate workers to be on time or behave more positively in general. Perhaps time off or some other benefit would have been more successful as a motivator. The work force needs to be consulted; after all, the workers are the ones who must respond to the program.

MOTIVATION IN THE HEALTH CARE SETTING

As management begins to struggle with the development of a motivational program and attempts to decide on a suitable assessment tool, a number of important factors need to be considered. Twelve key factors emerged from two major research projects that examined the attitudes of health care workers and the factors that made them satisfied with their jobs. Eight hundred workers were surveyed in a two-year period with the use of the *Health Workers' Attitude Inventory.*[5] The factors emerging from this questioning suggest what is important to health care workers, and they can be used as the basis for critiquing, developing or selecting an assessment tool for determining what factors motivate the workers in a particular institution.

Although the factors are broad and the list is by no means comprehensive, the reader should nevertheless benefit from an improved understanding of the complexity of the forces that actually motivate a group of workers. These factors can be used as the basis for developing a tailor-made program or for generating a list of questions or issues when attempting to motivate the work force.

1. Input. Workers want the opportunity to speak up about their jobs. They want the chance to suggest change and

to perceive that they are heard by management and supervision. In the studies this was a particularly strong concern of RNs.

2. Worker–supervisor relations. The supervisor is the key to organizational harmony and the success of motivational programs. Supervisors must know how to accomplish their jobs and how to be fair, understanding, mature and helpful. In the studies this factor was a particularly strong concern of RNs and allied health professionals.

The supervisor is the key to organizational harmony and the success of motivational programs.

3. Discipline/grievance. Workers desire policies and procedures that are fair and unbiased. Policy and procedure can act as powerful motivators.

4. Work environment. The environment has to be perceived as clean, comfortable and safe. These items often emerge as particular concerns of housekeeping personnel and allied health professionals.

5. Breaks and meals. Workers feel the need for time off during working hours. Breaking away appears essential to RNs, who often get little or no time to rest because of staffing situations.

6. Discrimination. Workers of all job classifications display a general aversion to racial, sexual and professional discrimination. Fairness in this dimension is highly critical and is more of an issue for female workers than for male workers.

7. Job satisfaction. Workers will be motivated if they have jobs that make them feel good about themselves. Individuals need to feel they have a future in the organization, and their work load must be perceived as reasonable. This dimension presents a particular challenge for the supervisor in areas where workers have limited upward mobility because of training or educational constraints.

8. Performance appraisals. The formal appraisal sessions and faithful follow-up are vital parts of an ongoing motivational program. One must also recognize the value and impact of informal appraisal sessions and balance their use with the use of formal procedures. Appraisal and feedback must occur on a regular and timely basis and must be equitable. Supervisors must be thoroughly trained in appraisal methods. If all appropriate factors are not considered, a performance appraisal may have a negative impact on the individuals involved.

9. Clarity of policy, procedure and benefits. Workers must understand and possess *working* knowledge of policy and procedure and particularly of their benefits. Often workers are not highly motivated because supervisors fail to do a thorough job of explaining all the benefits of employment. It is the supervisor's responsibility to serve as a teacher and a resource person in this area. Sick leave, vacation, health insurance and maternity benefits are invariably of particular concern and value as motivators.

10. Pay and development opportunities. Workers want pay that is fair in comparison with the pay of competing health care institutions and with the community in general. Other employers outside of the health care system cannot be ignored. Nurses are particularly concerned about development opportunities, including both continuing education and the opportunity to grow within the organization.

11. Decision making. Workers want something to say about how the institution or agency is managed; they want to experience a true vested interest. This dimension has been shown to be especially important to RNs and allied health professionals.

12. Style of management. The attitude workers perceive that top management projects through

the individual supervisors is an important factor. Health care workers want to be associated with an organization that cares about workers and patients alike. Beyond this, however, workers do not want to be ignored; they desire a fair and consistent style of management.

TAKING ACTION

Once there has been an assessment by the organization of the workers' perceptions, it remains for the supervisor to link the appropriate motivators to performance. The valued reward must be dispensed in the appropriate fashion. Feedback must be accurate and timely and participation must be encouraged whenever it is possible to do so.

This approach to motivation and reward cannot be a one-time event. Attitudes must be assessed formally on a regular basis, preferably every six to nine months. Beyond applying formal measures the supervisor must constantly monitor the worker's feelings through open communication.

Supervisors must be ever aware that even the best program in the world will not be effective without their conscientious commitment and active effort. Also, administrators must accept their responsibility to train first-line and middle-level supervisors in how to do their jobs effectively and efficiently.

The motivation for supervisors must lie always in remembering that worker performance is the key to their own performance, and that understanding worker perceptions is thus the key to effective supervision.

REFERENCES

1. Levine, H.A. "Efforts to Improve Productivity." *Personnel* 60 (January/February 1983): 4–10.
2. Fitzgerald, P.E. "Developing the Health Workers' Attitude Inventory: A Tool for Assessing Worker/Management Relations in Health Care Institutions." Dissertation, University of Alabama in Birmingham, March 1982.
3. McCreight, R.E. "A Five Role System for Motivating Improved Performance." *Personnel Journal* 62 (January 1983): 30.
4. Levine, H.A. "Efforts to Improve Productivity."
5. Fitzgerald, "Developing the Health Workers' Attitude Inventory."

Part II
The Supervisor and the Employee

Employee clout: "who's running this organization, anyway?"

Charles R. McConnell
Vice President for Employee Affairs
The Genesee Hospital
Rochester, New York

DURING ONE sample month of 1983, in a particular health care organization, the following occurred:

- Eleven employees were separated from the organization. Four of them were discharged—two for gross misconduct, one for insubordination, and one for a severe attendance problem (failing to show up for work and failing to call in as required by policy, for three consecutive days). Six employees resigned voluntarily, citing a range of reasons—to take other employment, to leave the work force altogether, to relocate to another area, and simply to resign for "personal reasons." One employee was released shortly before the end of the probationary period for inability to meet the requirements of the job.
- Of the eleven separated employees, eight, each within one week of termination, filed for unem-

Health Care Superv, 1985,4(1),70–82
© 1985 Aspen Publishers, Inc.

ployment compensation. In the opinion of the organization's human resources department, only one of these eight employees—the one dismissed for inability to meet the requirements of the job—was entitled to unemployment compensation. The eight people who applied for unemployment compensation included three who had voluntarily resigned.

- One employee who was discharged for gross misconduct was a member of a recognized minority group and filed a discrimination complaint with the State Division of Human Rights. The complaint alleged that the discharge was prejudicial because of the individual's minority status.
- A female clerical worker visited the human resources department to complain of her male supervisor's language and of his "chauvinistic attitude." She made it plain that she was reasonably conversant with the laws that made the organization responsible for continuation of such behavior once it was reported to management, and she hinted that charges of sexual harassment might be forthcoming if nothing was done to change her work situation.
- A candidate for a technician position voluntarily revealed to the interviewing supervisor that she was pregnant. When she was not offered the position—she was

but one of several candidates, some of whom were more highly qualified—she filed a charge of sex discrimination with the State Division of Human Rights. Her complaint charged the interviewing supervisor with asking her if she was pregnant and then not hiring her because of this condition.

- A female employee who did not receive a promotion she strongly desired filed a lawsuit against the organization claiming damage to her career through sex discrimination. She had two years experience in the job and better-than-average performance evaluations; however, her attendance record was marginal. The employee who actually received the promotion—a male—likewise had two years experience and above-average performance evaluations, but his attendance record was near perfect. The female employee's attorney also filed a charge of sex discrimination with the Equal Employment Opportunity Commission (EEOC), which in turn resulted in automatic filing of a complaint of sex discrimination with the State Division of Human Rights.
- In addition to the foregoing, four other employees filed grievances according to the organization's internal grievance procedure.

The activities necessitated by the foregoing actions and complaints resulted in the following:

- The organization contested seven of the eight unemployment claims and received favorable determination on all seven. However, it was necessary to go through unemployment hearings before an administrative law judge in five of the seven cases. (Two of the former employees did not ask for hearings after the initial denial of benefits.) However, winning all seven unemployment cases consumed about 45 hours, with about 20 of these hours being spent by the supervisors of the former employees and the balance consumed by activities of the human resources department.
- The human rights complaint charging discrimination against a minority was dismissed on the basis of no probable cause. However, obtaining this determination required the organization to gather and submit significant amounts of information and participate in a field investigation of the complaint. Overall some 40 hours were consumed in internal effort, divided about equally between human resources and line supervision. There were also several hundred dollars in costs for legal guidance, and the entire process led to a supposedly routine no-probable-cause determination stretched out over nearly four calendar months.
- Human resources and line management took steps to deal with the informal sexual harassment complaint, working discreetly with the persons involved. This process required some 30 hours of effort, again about equally divided between human resources and line management, but a potentially costly and time-consuming formal complaint was avoided.
- The complaint of the pregnant job candidate also resulted in a no-probable-cause determination. However, the organization had to spend approximately 35 hours over the course of two months establishing that, first, this individual was not hired simply because there was a more qualified candidate available, and second, that the organization had indeed hired numerous applicants who happened to be pregnant solely because they were best suited for the positions for which they were applying.
- Regarding the lawsuit brought by the female employee who did not get the promotion she desired, after investigation a determination of no probable cause was rendered on the human rights complaint. There followed, after a considerable delay, a similar determination on the complaint submitted to the EEOC. Apparently because of these two determinations in favor of the organization, the lawsuit was dropped. Overall this case took approximately 100 hours and cost several thousand dollars in legal expenses.
- All four of the employee grievances were eventually settled,

two of them in favor of the complainants. For all four grievances the average settlement time came close to 20 hours each, with about 8 to 10 hours for each grievance spent by the complainants' immediate superiors.

A crude tally of the cost to the organization of accomplishing the foregoing resolutions, taking into account the major cost elements only (for example, no effort was made to estimate the cost of the considerable amounts of photocopying involved), showed these actions consumed about 165 hours of direct involvement of supervisors and middle managers, about an equal amount of time for the involvement of human resources professionals, and the expenditure of several thousand dollars in out-of-pocket costs.

Thus it may seem to many supervisors and managers that much of their time and an appreciable amount of the organization's resources, rather than being devoted to getting out the work, are consumed in dealing with the problems presented by employees. As one supervisor who was involved in two of the foregoing complaints observed, "I'm spending more time listening to employees who are trying to tell me what to do than I am in legitimately listening to *management* telling me what to do. Who's running this organization, anyway?"

A BALANCE OF POWER

Prior to 1964 there were essentially no major avenues of legal recourse for

With minor exceptions—workers' compensation, unemployment compensation, and the like—before 1964 matters concerned with conditions of employment were largely unregulated for the majority of health care organizations.

health care employees outside of their employing organizations. Although business organizations of all kinds were subject to far less outside intervention in employee matters before 1964, health care organizations were even less affected than other businesses and industries. Before 1964, for example, most other kinds of organizations had to be fully responsive to the Fair Labor Standards Act (FLSA); however, not-for-profit hospitals were exempt from the minimum wage and overtime requirements of the FLSA. Also, other businesses and industries were subject to the National Labor Relations Act (NLRA), but this legislation did not yet apply to not-for-profit health care organizations. Thus with minor exceptions—workers' compensation, unemployment compensation, and the like—before 1964 matters concerned with conditions of employment were largely unregulated for the majority of health care organizations. Since the early sixties, however, the following have taken place:

- Title VI of the Civil Rights Act of 1964 prohibited discrimination based on race, color, or national origin in all programs or activities receiving federal financial aid. Already affected, then, were health care organizations that had used federal grant money for building and expansion. The prohibitions of Title VI came into full force in 1966 when the federal government became fully involved in health care funding through Medicare and Medicaid.

- Title VII of the Civil Rights Act of 1964, and especially as later amended by the Equal Employment Opportunity Act of 1972, prohibited discrimination because of race, color, religion, sex, or national origin in any term, condition, or privilege of employment.
- Executive Order 11246, issued in 1965, required affirmative action programs by all federal contractors and subcontractors, requiring that organizations with contracts over $50,000 and 50 or more employees develop and implement written programs to be monitored by an assigned compliance agency. For many organizations this essentially mandated affirmative action plans and brought under scrutiny many organizations' patterns of minority and female employment.
- The Equal Pay Act of 1963 required all employers subject to the Fair Labor Standards Act to provide equal pay for men and women performing similar work. This is significant largely in light of the following item.
- During 1967 the Fair Labor Stan-

dards Act was amended to call for the application of minimum wage and overtime requirements equally in not-for-profit hospitals as in other industries.

- The Age Discrimination in Employment Act of 1967 prohibited all employers of twenty or more persons from discriminating against persons in the forty- to seventy-year-old age range in any area of employment strictly because of age.
- In 1975 the National Labor Relations Act was amended to remove the exemption of not-for-profit hospitals. By removing this specific exemption that had been in effect since 1947, it became legally possible for unions to organize workers in not-for-profit health care organizations.

In addition to the foregoing there have been other pieces of legislation affecting the employment practices of some health care organizations, including, for example, the Education Amendments Act of 1972, the Rehabilitation Act of 1973, the Vietnam Veterans Readjustment Assistance Act of 1974, and various state and local laws.

In addition to myriad legislation and the creation of a number of government agencies to which employees with problems can turn, employees have also been exposed to significant amounts of information in the public press and other public forums concerning individual rights. Television reports, newspaper stories, and magazine articles have made many persons keenly aware of such things as their legal rights regarding practices such as sexual harassment; the progressive erosion of the age-old concept of employment-at-will (the notion that an employee serves at the convenience of the employer and can be discharged at any time for no stated reason); and, successful age discrimination lawsuits that have been brought by persons who were separated from employment against their will during their middle years.

Also present today, but not a factor twenty years or so ago, are a variety and number of social action agencies, generally voluntary, not-for-profit advocacy groups formed to advance the causes of minority groups and others of certain common interests. Many such organizations frequently provide advice and encouragement to individuals who feel they were wronged and show these people how to file complaints with various agencies and how in general to use the elements of the system that are available for their benefit.

Another factor in the increasing frequency of employee actions against present and former employers is to be found in the changing nature of society. In these days of increasing consciousness of the rights of the individual, fewer people are willing to tolerate actions that they might consider unjust. Society is becoming increasingly litigious; today more than ever before it is easier to say "I'll sue" and turn to members of the legal profession.

By and large, today's employees are far more knowledgeable about their rights than their counterparts of two or three decades ago. Today's employees, educated and armed with information, are quick to discover that a growing number of channels of recourse are open to them. Thus the employee who feels that he or she has been wronged by an employing organization may file a complaint according to the organization's grievance procedure, file a legal complaint with any of a number of federal, state, and local government agencies, or engage an attorney and initiate a lawsuit.

A comparison of the health care organization of the early 1960s with its counterpart of today thoroughly confirms that in the past the employee with a perceived complaint essentially stood alone against the organization. The power was all in the hands of the organization; for the most part, any employee could be reassigned, demoted, or discharged at the will of the organization and could in some ways even be regularly treated in a manner that many would now legitimately consider to be abusive.

Today, one need only listen to a representative group of supervisors and human resources professionals tell of their experiences with actions brought by aggrieved employees to know that the 1980s atmosphere presents far more difficulties for both individual supervisors and their employing organizations. In the past, many supervisors could behave either carelessly or callously or both and get away with it. Now, the supervisor who behaves carelessly or callously runs a high risk of triggering a legal action that can result in much frustrating, time-consuming activity, and considerable expense to the organization. Certainly many of today's supervisors are willing to express the belief that individual employees—including many whose grievances are without merit—are able to intimidate and manipulate entire organizations almost at will.

One might even occasionally wonder if the balance of power has shifted completely from the organization to the individual. This thought may seem ludicrous at first; however, from the perspective of the individual supervisor it might often appear that the individual employee is pushing the organization around. Certainly individual employees, even those whose complaints are without merit, can cause the organization some extra work and some added expense. However, when it comes to pushing the organization around, those employees who eventually have such impact are usually able to do so because of a legal determination in their favor—that is, they happen to be "right."

Thus it is not a complete swing of the power balance that has taken place; rather, what has occurred is more of an equalization of the ability to engage in a search for an appropriate solution to a perceived difference. It is no longer the lone person against the organization. Now the individual who has been wronged or who perceives that he or she has been wronged has advocates and has active

assistance in pursuing resolution. From the point of view of the person, no longer is it a hopelessly one-sided situation of "me" versus "all of them"; rather, it is now more nearly a matter of "us" against "them."

THE SUPERVISOR'S ALTERED ROLE

Before 1964 the individual supervisors or managers had far more freedom to act as they may have seen fit in any particular situation. Certainly many work organizations have long used standard procedures for parceling out disciplinary action and for terminating employees. However, for a variety of reasons, such procedures were not always necessarily followed; but the fact that they were not followed meant little—in the majority of cases there was no great risk involved and no penalty associated with not following procedure. For the most part a supervisor could safely adopt an attitude reflecting "This is my department, and I'll run it the way I see fit." In all fairness to many supervisors of past years, the way one chose to "see fit" might have been fair, humane, and impartial. Just as readily, however, the supervisor's approach could have in some way been arbitrary, as the supervisor may have acted against some employees out of personality considerations or out of personal bias.

This is certainly not to say that deliberate discrimination was always at the heart of most supervisors' actions toward employees. It is even more likely that a significant number of essentially unjust personnel actions stemmed from thoughtlessness, carelessness, and inconsistency on the part of supervisors. In short, supervisors' actions tended to be loose and inconsistent because there were no external pressures on the organization to encourage supervisors and managers to behave in any other way.

Now, however, there are numerous restrictions on the behavior of supervisors in their dealings with employees. These are legal requirements placed on the supervisor's employing organization, but they instantly translate to requirements on the individual supervisor who, in most matters involving the employment relationship, is acting as an agent of the organization. The organization ultimately bears responsibility for the actions of its supervisors, but it is reasonable to assume that the supervisor who commits an infraction that brings discredit or penalty to the organization will likely become the object of some organizational criticism or disciplinary action.

Surely there are a number of reasons for today's health care supervisors, especially those who have been in their positions for a number of years, to feel increasing frustration in working with troublesome employees. In most organizations, supervisors have encountered an increasing amount of involvement in their employee problems by the human resources department. Although this involvement may be viewed as necessary to achieve legally consis-

It is understandable that supervisors may view the human resources function as interfering—telling them what to do in matters that were once exclusively within their own province.

tent employee treatment throughout the organization, it is understandable that supervisors may view the human resources function as interfering—telling them what to do in matters that were once exclusively within their own province. Thus supervisors, already feeling, as many have felt for years, that employee problems are a definite intrusion on their basic responsibility of getting the work done, are frequently led to see the human resources function as an unwelcome intrusion on how they handle their people problems. Human resources—still *personnel* in the minds of many—seems constantly to be telling them what they should be doing when they are doing nothing, and what they cannot do when they are doing something.

Within a scant quarter of a century the individual supervisor has made the transition from being able to deal with employee problems fully, freely, and independently, to being forced to react to a significant number of constraints and restrictions in such dealings. Today's rank and file employees do indeed have clout in a number of matters, so much clout that a supervisor is forced to thoroughly analyze all aspects of any given employment action before it is implemented. In the face of such employee clout there seem to be but two ultimate directions in which the supervisor can go: The supervisor can drift in passive directions, caving in under employee pressure and avoiding even the possibility of complaints, and, for those circumstances that do eventually emerge as complaints, allow human resources and administration to call the shots; or the supervisor can take an active role in practicing modern employee relations. If it is doing nothing else positive, the genuine employee clout prevalent today is at least forcing many supervisors to sharpen their managerial skills and to focus considerably more attention on the all-important supervisor–employee relationship.

COUNTERING EMPLOYEE CLOUT

As previously suggested, it may presently seem that individual employees actually have the upper hand in the employment arrangement. However, this is not the case; employees, who for years were on the short end of the employment relationship when trouble arose, have simply achieved, through law, a more nearly equal footing with the organization. This suggests that even though there are specific processes that can be activated when an employee feels wronged by the organization, so are there processes to be employed by the supervisor and the organization when an employee seems not to be appropriately fulfilling the employment relationship. There are several ways in which the supervisor can become better able to deal with employee problems of today. In addition to knowing and using the organization's human resources function, the supervisor can learn the organization's personnel policies and reassess his or her interviewing skills. Also, supervisors may deal with problems by generating objective performance appraisals, by using the progressive disciplinary process, and by viewing employee conduct and employee performance separately.

The human resources function

The human resources department represents a classic staff function. It is not part of the line organization—it delivers no patient care and it generates no income. Therefore, as a pure staff function it exists for one purpose—to provide service to the rest of the organization, employees and managers alike. As with any staff function, one might be able to argue that the organization could operate, after a fashion, without this activity, but clearly the organization will run much better with this particular function. The key word of course is *service*. As a service function, human resources is there to serve the supervisor.

Supervisors should take advantage of the human resources function. Human resources is usually a provider of current information about what can or cannot legally be done in any employment situation. This department ordinarily has a direct pipeline to legal advice on questions that cannot be immediately dealt with in-house. When the supervisor takes employee relations problems—and suggested solutions, if any—to human resources, he or she will generally encounter benefits of two kinds: knowledge will be obtained of what is or is not likely to be possible under law, framed in a way that enhances organization-wide consistency; and, information will be absorbed about today's employee problems that will serve later, in situations not yet encountered.

Personnel policies

Surely most health care organizations operating in the current environment endeavor to maintain thorough, up-to-date personnel policies. In light of continually changing conditions it might even be said that absolutely complete and current personnel policies represent a goal to be always sought but never fully achieved. Regardless of completeness, however, chances are that the organization's personnel policies deal with many matters of concern in the employment relationship. The supervisor should study the organization's personnel policies and should try to apply them as he or she under-

stands them. Further, the supervisor should challenge those aspects of policy that appear to be incomplete or that seem not to provide the means for dealing thoroughly with the situations being encountered. It is only through information supplied by all active policy-using supervisors that the organization can keep its personnel policies truly up-to-date.

Reassessment of interviewing skills

Often the employee selection interview is a source of employee problems of two kinds: The conduct and performance problems that can result if the candidate selected is not the "right" person for the job; and, the problems that come in the form of complaints from persons who claim they were not hired because they were discriminated against in the employment process.

In general, the interviewing supervisor can ask no questions that could be construed as soliciting information concerning an applicant's age, marital status, race, religion, national origin, or general economic status. For example, it is generally inappropriate to even ask if the applicant owns a home or an automobile because this may be interpreted as seeking to test affluence, and may in turn be taken as discriminatory against certain minorities. Asking if the applicant has a driver's license is advisable only if driving is a *bona fide occupational requirement* (BFOR); that is, a requirement of the job. Generally, the supervisor is on the firmest footing in questioning a prospective employee when all questions of a personal nature relate only to legitimate requirements of the job. Again, the human resources department should be seen as the source of information and guidance on how selection should be done. In many organizations, human resources will (or should) offer periodic instruction for supervisors on how to interview job applicants.

The organization as a whole must be extremely careful in asking prospective employees for information. Much that is needed for employment purposes, such as birth date, names and ages of spouse and children, can legally be requested only after an individual has accepted a job offer. If an organization's employment application is older than five years, it may well include illegal elements. The human resources department must ensure that the employment application is consistent with present law.

Objective performance appraisals

Many of the problems supervisors face in dealing with matters of employee misconduct and substandard performance cannot reasonably be dealt with as they should because proposed actions are not supported by appropriate documentation of the past. It is not unusual for an occasional supervisor to reach a position of finally having had it with an employee who is considered substandard or, at best, marginal. Yet when the supervisor finally decides to eliminate the supposedly substandard em-

ployee, the employee's personnel file reveals a series of standard or satisfactory evaluations.

Certainly it is easier to rate a marginal or slightly substandard employee as standard and thus avoid all of the hassles that may be associated with justifying a rating that may be partly subjective, and taking additional steps to bring the employee up to expectations. However, the longer one carries a substandard performer the harder it becomes to do anything about that employee. When government agencies become involved in employment disputes—and when they do, the personnel file is generally requested by legal means—outside agencies have no choice but to accept ratings of standard or average at face value. An employee who in the supervisor's best judgment and according to all evaluation criteria appears to be performing at substandard levels should be rated accordingly. Rarely can a contention of substandard past performance be supported when the record says otherwise.

Progressive discipline

There are a few possible infractions of work rules that traditionally call for discharge on occurrence of the first and only offense. These include falsification of time records, fighting or otherwise physically assaulting another person, insubordination, theft, and other instances of gross misconduct. However, the majority of infractions that may be committed by an employee are considered to merit only a warning and some counseling, and an opportunity for the employee to correct the inappropriate behavior. In most instances—all but cases of gross misconduct clearly identified in policy—the outside agencies that monitor the organization's employment actions will attempt to answer one specific question: Was the employee given ample opportunity to correct the inappropriate behavior? This approach is advanced on the generally held belief that the primary purpose of disciplinary action should be correction of behavior. Thus if the organization's policy states, relative to a certain type of infraction, that counseling should take place and that two warnings of increasing severity should follow if behavior does not improve, after which discharge may take place, in any specific case the supervisor and the organization may be called on to produce the paper trail of the progressive discipline. This process—the thorough, conscientious application of the organization's progressive discipline procedure—is one of the supervisor's strongest defenses against employee complaints of mistreatment.

Conduct versus performance

Matters of conduct, those instances of violation of the organization's work rules, are most appropriately handled through the progressive disciplinary procedure. However, matters of employee performance are not as appropriately handled through this same procedure. When an employee breaks a work rule, the disciplinary process deals with the employee's knowledge of that particular rule. However, when the employee's problem is performance related, for example, failing to meet the quantity or quality standard of the job, then more than ever the supervisor is likely to come under close scrutiny concerning the opportunities the employee may or may not have been given to learn the appropriate ways of doing things. Thus an employee problem that develops around performance will ordinarily be addressed through counseling sessions that provide the employee with clearly understandable objectives for improvement in particular job functions, perhaps accompanied by extra orientation or additional job-related instruction. It is only after all reasonable—and provable—steps have been taken to bring performance up to standard that a substandard employee should be released. Also, an employee released due to an inability to meet the standards of the job is sometimes not considered *fired* so much as *laid off*—that is, unable to do the job—and so will often be eligible for unemployment compensation.

● ● ●

In these days of increasing employment regulation it is necessary for the supervisor to become as familiar as possible with all of the applicable elements of law affecting the employment relationship. Although much of what has herein been described as employee clout may appear as an unwelcome change in the way the supervisory job must be accomplished, by and large it represents permanent change. In one important respect, regulation of employment is much like regulation of the organization's financial life—it is highly likely that the future will bring more, not less, regulation. To one who might ask in frustration, "Who's running this organization, anyway?," the response might be: Management—from the chief executive officer down to and including each individual supervisor—is still running the organization. The task has simply become a bit more demanding and considerably more challenging.

The visible supervisor

Charles R. McConnell
Vice President for Employee Affairs
The Genesee Hospital
Rochester, New York

"IF THE BOSS CALLS, GET HIS NAME"

IN THE BOOK *Up the Organization* there is a revealing checklist titled "Rate Your Boss as a Leader."[1] Author Townsend, in two of the list's ten points, describes a good boss as "objective. Knows the apparently important (like a visiting director) from the truly important (a meeting of his own people) and goes where he is needed." A good boss is also "available. If I have a problem I can't solve, he is there."

An important notion for supervisors to consider is how high they would score if their employees rated them on these two points. On a scale of zero ("Boss? *What* boss?") to ten ("a Saint!"), how well would supervisors fare in employees' assessments of their visibility and availability? If a supervisor has serious doubts about his or her likely score, perhaps it is time for that supervisor to reexamine the importance of management visibility and reconsider the need to be available to his or her employees.

The quotation in the heading came from an accountant in the finance group of a large medical center. He saw his manager, the vice president for finance, once or twice a week, if that often. He felt he knew his job well, but more often than he might have cared to admit, he encountered situations requiring knowledge beyond his capabilities or calling for the exercise of authority he did not possess. He was not bashful about taking on problems that were over his head, and often his solutions were appropriate. Just as often, however, he was wrong, but he became fairly adept at shrugging off the consequences. It was usually while plunging into the latest panic, after attempts to reach the vice president had failed, that he was likely to say, "If the boss calls, get his name."

Challenge and growth were aspects of many situations the accountant faced. However, other elements were often present as well: helplessness, frustration and a sense of being let down in a pinch.

Supervisors are busy people. Supervisors who try to do a good job while advancing their careers are likely to find the demands on their time far exceeding their supply of time. In the face of conflicting demands, something will get their attention, and something will suffer. Too often the wrong "something" can

be allowed to command the quality portion of supervisors' time and effort.

FACING UPWARD OR DOWNWARD IN AN ORGANIZATION

Supervisors and other managers are middle-of-the-organization workers. Except for those at the very top, they report to other managers. Since they also have employees who report to them, most supervisors experience demands from below as well as from above. These demands are felt as pressures to "face downward" toward employees and their problems and needs, and pressures to "face upward" toward higher management.

The pressures causing supervisors to face upward are undeniable: direct orders, requests of other managers and opportunities to make themselves visible outside of their limited areas and thus enhance their organizational standing. The usually absent vice president referred to earlier was always doing *something* related to his work—he was at an interdepartmental meeting, serving on a committee, sitting in *his* boss's office, attending a conference or seminar outside of the hospital or developing a budget or writing a report.

Supervisors cannot be blamed for wanting to be noticed by higher management and others who control or influence promotions and other rewards. There is an old saying, "The boss ain't always right, but the boss is always the boss." A manager who rose in the organization with an up-ward-facing orientation may uncon-sciously seek this same orientation in potential subordinate managers. Fac-ing upward may sometimes seem the way for a supervisor to get ahead; however, it will usually only help him or her to move up a notch or two in the organization, and it is of no value whatsoever if the supervisor's immediate superior rightly places people, output and organizational goals ahead of self-interest.

For supervisors the greatest hazard in facing upward—in the direction, supposedly, of status and recogni-

---

For supervisors the greatest hazard in facing upward—in the direction, supposedly, of status and recognition—is the likelihood of losing sight of those immediately below them in the organization.

---

tion—is the likelihood of losing sight of those immediately below them in the organization. Employees ulti-mately have the greatest effect on the performance of supervisors, but it is all too easy for supervisors to become so busy facing upward that they lose touch with the people who can truly make or break them.

"Absentee ownership" may work well in business when the arrange-ment includes strong on-site, day-to-day management. However, "absen-tee management," whether in a small

business or a department of a large institution, will not work. Many small hospitals, for instance, struggle along on absentee management. The pres-sures causing hospital administrators to face upward and outward are many: medical staff, boards of direc-tors, community, associations, com-missions and others.

In a small facility in which top management is a one-person show, something is bound to suffer. The irony of this situation is that the up-ward-and-outward-facing administra-tor is more likely to be noticed when desirable positions open up. The per-son who stays in his or her assigned area and concentrates on running an efficient organization is less visible to the industry and thus less likely to be recruited.

FACING THE REAL ACTION

Will a supervisor's department run satisfactorily most of the time without the supervisor, fueled by proper del-egation and clear standing orders? Only if the supervisor has an assist-ant, fully as knowledgeable and capa-ble as the supervisor and empowered to act on all matters in his or her ab-sence. If the outside pressures are sufficient to justify the arrangement, the supervisor and his or her assistant can act as an "outside-inside" team, with one relating to the rest of the organization and one "minding the store."

However, many supervisors and middle managers are not blessed with assistants; the scope of responsibility and limited amounts of legitimate upward-and-outward contact do not justify additional help. In this common situation, the supervisor is forced to wear both hats.

Regardless of proper delegation and standing orders, a department will not run as well *without* the supervisor as it can run *with* the supervisor. Much of the supervisor's job consists of *control* (follow-up and correction), solving operating problems, dealing with personnel problems and making hour-to-hour decisions in light of changing conditions and unforeseen circumstances. The supervisor must be there when the problems arise, or at least be readily available, to maintain proper control of the operation. It is not sufficient for the supervisor to leave a telephone number and say, "Call me if anything happens." If reaching the supervisor becomes difficult or time consuming, many problems that the supervisor should handle will never reach his or her attention. Even if the supervisor can be located if something disastrous occurs, his or her lack of visibility may prevent lesser but still important problems from reaching him or her. If employees must always go out of their way to pull the supervisor back to the department, after a while they simply will not bother to look for the supervisor. After all, if the supervisor seems not to care, why should *they* care?

Not being on hand to deal with day-to-day problems also represents a forfeiture of authority. A supervisor may avoid exercising the authority of his or her position by not being present to decide and act, but the *responsibility* for what goes on in that department remains the supervisor's. The full recognition of the implications of such responsibility as a fact of organizational life is often enough to encourage a supervisor to establish new priorities, especially when the supervisor begins to feel that he or she is drifting away from the employee group.

When a supervisor is not available, many questions and problems that should be brought to management's attention never get heard. When the accountant in the example introduced earlier could not find his absentee manager, much of the time he took some risks and made decisions he was neither qualified nor authorized to make. Other times he ignored the problems and hoped they would go away. On one occasion the institution suffered a costly reimbursement penalty because of one "small" problem the accountant ignored. The vice president was unhappy with the accountant, but that was nothing compared with how unhappy the president was with the vice president.

THE EMPLOYEE'S VIEW

Every supervisor should occasionally ask, "Right now, how am I likely to be viewed by my employees?" If there are any doubts connected with the answer, the next question should be, "How much of my time and attention did I give my employees today?"

A supervisor is in a unique position relative to the people who report to him or her. The supervisor may be the only member of that mysterious entity called "management" that employees know on a speaking basis. It is likely that the supervisor is the individual employee's sole channel of communication with administration and the primary point of contact with the rest of the organization. If employees regard a supervisor as distant, unavailable, uncaring, and lacking time for them—all impressions created by a management style that emphasizes facing upward—so may they also come to regard the institution as a whole. In short, as employees view the supervisor, so also are they likely to view the organization.

The importance of the employee's view of the supervisor is illustrated in the following case situation, which deals with the supervisor's availability and visibility. The employee viewpoint was deliberately used in the case description to make a point: The supervisor may feel that he or she is appropriately visible to employees—plural—but it is only what is seen by a single employee that determines that particular employee's view of the supervisor.

IN SEARCH OF THE FAST-MOVING BOSS: AN ILLUSTRATION

The problem

Roger J., a purchasing agent at a large city hospital, reported to Harry R., the Manager of Materiel Manage-

ment. Roger long felt that the greatest area of frustration in his job was his relationship with his supervisor. Specifically, it was Harry's availability— or rather, extremely limited availability—that most confounded Roger. Roger believed that he was fully capable of doing his job with limited supervision, but he also believed that he required *some* supervision. He was especially concerned with instances in which he felt pressured to act beyond the limits of his authority on matters in which his supervisor should clearly have been involved.

After several occasions of feeling at risk for making decisions that should probably have had Harry's stamp of approval, Roger decided that the next time such an occasion arose he would keep a record of his attempts to involve Harry. The following Monday morning when Roger was faced with a problem that promised to strain the limits of his authority, he began to document his efforts to reach Harry. Relative to Harry and the problem, Roger's week proceeded as follows:

Monday. Roger telephoned Harry's office four times throughout the day. Each time, Harry's secretary said he was "busy" and that she would leave word for him to call back. On his fourth call Roger left word that his need involved "a matter of considerable importance." However, Monday ended with no response from Harry.

Tuesday. By pure chance Roger saw Harry coming toward him along a basement corridor. Stepping out so as to nearly block Harry's passage, Roger said, "I've got a hot one, Harry.

We need to get together." Without slowing, Harry detoured around Roger and called back over his shoulder, "Got a hot one myself, can't stop, get back with you in a little bit." Harry did not call, nor did Roger see him again that day. Roger telephoned Harry's office but was told that Harry was in a meeting.

Wednesday. In the morning Roger decided to make an unannounced visit to Harry's office. However, he discovered that Harry had two visitors. Harry saw Roger through the glass of the office door and shrugged, smiled faintly and waved Roger away. In the afternoon Roger again tried telephoning Harry. After several rings Harry answered his own phone, immediately explained that he was tied up with an important visitor and added, "Buzz you back as soon as I'm free." Roger remained at work well after quitting time, but Harry did not call back. When Roger left for the day, he noticed that Harry's parking space was already empty.

Thursday. Roger made but one attempt to contact Roger—an unsuccessful telephone call. The item he had been holding open since Monday was crying for a decision, so Roger gave in and made the decision. He was sure that he was overstepping his authority, but he was certain that continued delay would only cause more trouble. Roger felt that he could perhaps hedge his decision to some extent, since it could be reversed without harm anytime before the end of Friday.

Friday. Roger encountered Harry twice while moving about the base-

ment level of the hospital. The first time Roger said that he needed a few minutes of Harry's time "on the same hot item I've been trying to reach you about all week." Harry said that he was on his way to the administrator's office but that he would call Roger before noon. Noon came and went without a call. On the second occasion Harry saw Roger first and called out, "Hey, Roger, we need to get together, I'm on my way to an administrative staff meeting right now, but you can catch me in my office at 4:00." Harry was not in his office at 4:00 P.M., and he did not return during the 15 minutes Roger waited. Harry was not there at 4:30 P.M., when Roger returned, nor was he there at 5:00 P.M., when Roger made a final check before leaving for the weekend. On the way out of the building Roger learned that the administrative staff meeting had ended at 3:30.

During a few quiet moments at home, Roger reviewed his brief notes of the week and summarized his efforts to meet with Harry as follows:

1. Telephoned seven times.
   a. Six calls not returned.
   b. One direct contact; promised call not forthcoming.
2. Met by chance three times.
   a. Two promised calls not forthcoming.
   b. One promised meeting not made.
3. Visited office four times.
   a. One brief visual contact.
   b. Three times, office was empty.

By telephoning, visiting Harry's office and taking advantage of chance encounters, Roger made no fewer than 14 attempts to speak with his supervisor. He further reckoned that he

---

By telephoning, visiting Harry's office and taking advantage of chance encounters, Roger made no fewer than 14 attempts to speak with his supervisor.

---

had spent a total of nearly two hours—5 percent of his workweek—in unsuccessful attempts to secure a brief audience with his boss. Roger's work time was important to him, but worrying him even more than the time he lost because of Harry's behavior was the exposure he felt when he acted beyond the limits of his authority because Harry was unavailable.

The employee's options

If one assumes that the frustrating week sampled from Roger's working life is typical of the ongoing relationship between him and his supervisor, it appears that two options are available to Roger.

1. He may implement an all-out effort to get his boss's attention and try to establish some acceptable lines of communication.
2. He may go his own way without supervisory guidance, handling all problems that happen to come his way and generally accepting the risks involved in sometimes acting beyond the limits of his authority.

The first option, getting and keeping his boss's attention, is likely to require constant and determined effort on Roger's part. Many employees who have found themselves in similar circumstances have actually gone the way of the second option by default. Employees who find themselves in this latter position must usually be concerned with each individual problem until it forces action of some kind, disappears on its own or grows into a larger problem. Although more readily implemented because it requires no active effort, the second option is risky for the individual and carries the potential for considerably more harm to the organization.

To implement his first option, Roger might consider several methods. He could attempt to determine if there is any repeating pattern in Harry's seemingly limited availability and adjust to that pattern insofar as possible. For instance, if Roger is able to discover that Harry is in his office at 8:00 A.M. every day and that things are relatively quiet until 8:30 or so, he might safely conclude that 8:00 to 8:30 may be a good time to catch Harry for a moment's contact.

There may be other times—just before lunch, immediately after lunch, the last half-hour of the workday, or just before or just after some regularly scheduled meeting—that Roger might discover are opportune for speaking to Harry. Should he discover some times at which Harry seems to be more readily available, Roger should be prepared to arrange his own availability around Harry's.

Roger should be thorough in his contacts, taking answers and solutions, rather than questions and problems, to Harry. A supervisor usually has enough problems to worry about without each employee regularly bringing more. Instead of going to the boss and saying, "I have a problem— what shall I do?", it pays to do some homework and think the problem through and try to recommend at least an approach to a solution. When he does reach Harry with a problem, Roger should be saying, in effect: "I have a problem, here is why I think it's a problem, here are my possible solutions, here is the solution I think is best and why I think it's best, and here is my best assessment of what I need from you." The supervisor is not there to solve the employee's problem as much as to provide the information or authority needed to facilitate the solution.

Roger should consider relying on documentation to a considerable extent, putting in writing a great many things that might not necessarily be written if Harry were more visible or available. There are several helpful features of such a documentation approach. The approach uses specific questions that require brief, specific answers. For instance, if Roger sends Harry a memo or leaves him a note that describes a problem and potential solution and asks, "Is this what we should do?", Harry may be able to respond simply with "yes" or "no."

Some matters, well thought out as previously suggested, can be put in writing in such a way that nonre-sponse serves as consent. Roger may describe a problem and its suggested solution in a memo and add, "We need to resolve this by noon Wednesday. If I don't hear from you by then, I'll go ahead and take care of it." This approach can be risky at times, and if Roger is thinking ahead, he will allow a day or so of slack before taking action, simply to guard against the likelihood of a late response.

Roger may also want to send copies of some of his memos to other managers. Other members of management, Harry's peers, may have an interest in the problem. They will then know about it, and Harry will know that they know about it. However, Roger should be careful about including Harry's boss in the distribution of copies, since this action could be interpreted as an attempt to overstep his immediate supervisor. Roger may decide to send a copy to Harry's boss only when he is quite certain of his position and the matter is indeed critical.

When the use of documentation works at its best, Roger will find that he receives answers on a timely basis. If the best results are not forthcoming, in many instances Roger may at least find that he has protected himself by going on record as recognizing the problem and proposing a solution.

TWO IMPORTANT VIEWS

It is reasonable to suggest that most supervisors should be able to identify to some extent with Roger and Harry.

Like Harry, they have employees who report to them and depend on them for much communication. They are also in Roger's position in that they have bosses on whom they must depend for much of the support and assistance they need in accomplishing their jobs. It may aid supervisors' understanding of the positions in which supervisor and employee find themselves to briefly examine the views of both parties.

Looking upward

A supervisor may examine the implications of the communications environment from Roger's point of view; that is, from the point of view of the employee, recognizing that this is also the supervisor's point of view for examining relations with his or her boss. From the employee position, the supervisor is likely to see just one boss, one specific "source of help."

The supervisor sees the boss as being there to enable him or her to better accomplish his or her work for the benefit of the institution and its patients. It follows that the supervisor may feel frustration when that single source of assistance and support cannot be readily tapped when needed. However, the supervisor may not fully appreciate the reality of being just one of perhaps numerous subordinates who are likely to be placing demands on the time of the manager. Roger, for example, was but one of eight persons reporting directly to Harry.

Looking downward

Looking toward the employee group, the supervisor does not see a single point of contact. Rather, the supervisor sees as many sources of potential trouble and problems as there are employees. In the illustration Harry sees significantly more than Roger and his problem; Harry sees perhaps eight sources of problems, eight origins of demands on his time. It is likely that Roger's needs will often—even legitimately—take a back seat to certain other demands on Harry's time. It may seem overwhelming to the supervisor to be simultaneously aware of so many sources of demands, but the supervisor needs to realize that these apparent sources are very often points of true need.

Ideally, the supervisor and employee should appreciate each other's positions, accept each other's viewpoints and work to make it as easy as possible for each to communicate with the other. As suggested earlier, in the illustration Roger could take a number of steps to facilitate improved communications with Harry. However, most of the responsibility for enhanced communication lies with Harry—Harry is the supervisor in this relationship, and a larger share of the communication responsibility goes with the supervisory territory. Our illustration suggests that Harry has problems with visibility and availability. It would be helpful for Harry, as it would be for any supervisor experiencing similar difficulties, to take some active steps aimed at increasing visibility and improving availability.

HOW TO INCREASE VISIBILITY

The supervisor must learn to tell the truly important from the apparently important and go where the action is—or rather *stay* where the action is, since most of what is important in the fulfillment of the supervisor's responsibilities happens in his or her own department. The supervisor should ask: "Right now, of all the things I have to do, which is most im-

---

The supervisor should ask: "Right now, of all the things I have to do, which is most important to this department?"

---

portant to this department?" Note the use of "important to *this department*," not "important *to me*."

Each employee should be considered as a whole person, not merely as a piece of animated production equipment. The health care supervisor is there to help employees solve problems, provide service to patients and produce results. The supervisor is there to answer questions, deal with complaints, squelch rumors and put fears and suspicions to rest. All these are reasons for the supervisor's existence—and reasons for the supervisor's presence or ready availability as well.

Supervisors should remember that their employees do not work *for* them so much as *with* them. It is the re-

sponsibility of supervisors to run interference for their employees so that the employees can do their jobs as efficiently as possible.

A supervisor should maintain a true open-door policy with his or her employees. Few supervisors have not said, "My door is always open." However, those words often represent more platitude than attitude. The supervisor's door may be physically open, but if the supervisor's attitude says, "I'm busy, and you'd better not stick your head in without an appointment," he or she may as well close and lock the door.

Since some employees will not come to a supervisor under even the best of conditions, the supervisor should go to them. If the supervisor's span of control presents difficulties because he or she has dozens of employees scattered over a large physical area, the supervisor should make frequent tours at random intervals. This may entail a great deal of walking, but a supervisor is responsible for his or her employees' output, so the traveling goes with the territory.

When opportunity and space permit, the supervisor should avoid being isolated from employees. The comfort and status of a private office are appealing, but the best place for a department's supervisor is usually somewhere in the area in which most of his or her employees work. It is of course important for the supervisor to be able to have privacy when he or she needs it, but it is fully as important for the supervisor to remain readily accessible.

The supervisor should cultivate an honest one-to-one relationship with each employee. Instruction, information, praise and even correction are all enhanced by immediacy. A compliment or bit of criticism delivered days after the fact loses much of its impact. Immediate feedback is one of the strongest motivating forces in the relationship between manager and employee.

GETTING THINGS DONE THROUGH PEOPLE

The management job is often described as *getting things done through people*. To get things done through those all-important people—employees—supervisors should (1) be visible and available, spending most of their time where they are really needed; (2) show concern for their employees' problems; (3) maintain an "open-door" attitude and (4) rely on immediate feedback to let all of their employees know exactly where they stand.

Earlier it was suggested that as employees view their supervisor, so are they likely to view the institution as a whole. This concept of a reflected impression can be rearranged to lend perspective to supervisors' understanding of the pressures encouraging them to face upward: It could be that *as a boss views a department—*especially its efficiency or productivity—*so is the boss also likely to view the department's supervisor.*

REFERENCE

1. Townsend, R. *Up the Organization* (New York: Fawcett World Library 1971) p. 181–182.

A supervisory challenge: the difficult employee

Joan F. Moore
Nursing Administration Consultant
Tucson, Arizona

DOES YOUR DEPARTMENT have a high employee turnover rate? Why are people leaving? How many individuals fall into the category of "difficult employees"? How many were terminated for unacceptable behavior this year? How many since you have been supervisor? How many employees have been promoted out of or requested to leave your department?

High turnover is a major problem in the health care industry, and much of this turnover may be due to ineffective supervision. It would be to the supervisor's and the health care organization's benefit to evaluate the supervisor's skills and methods of dealing with difficult employees and to analyze whether there is a better way.

Humans behave in response to unsatisfied needs; their behavior is a direct result of their pursuit of the satisfaction of those needs within the

Health Care Superv, 1983,1(3),12–16
© 1983 Aspen Publishers, Inc.

framework of a value system. Problems can arise when the individual's behavior is in conflict with the value system of the individual's environment.

In the work environment, problems can arise when the needs of the employee conflict with the goals or value system of the organization or management. Such conflict often causes the supervisor to regard the employee involved as difficult. When this happens, it is up to the supervisor to determine why the conflict exists and how it can be dealt with.

First, the supervisor should determine if there is a good "fit" between the employee and the work situation. Do the employee's needs and goals correspond with those of the department and organization? The organization's value system is reflected in the specified job requirements, job standards, operational policies and guidelines, and leadership and supervisory interrelationships. Making sure that the organization's value system and the employee's needs mesh requires a close review of the methods and skills used in managing the employee.

THE HUMANISTIC APPROACH

Influencing people in a positive way

Bennett suggests that the humanistic way of managing people is to influence people in a positive way.[1] He suggests that the "key for the supervisor is to recognize his own personal and emotional weaknesses, his own behavior, his own values and at the same time to confront, understand and learn to accept the value systems of others."[2]

In the past, the difficult employee has primarily been addressed in the negative, with rules for disciplining and punishing by using force, authority, threats, etc. Haimann invites today's supervisor to discipline for improvement—to motivate rather than demotivate—and to promote the release of human potential.[3] Haimann believes supervisors should think of discipline as "a condition in which there is orderliness, in which the members of an organization behave themselves sensibly and conduct themselves according to the standards of acceptable behavior as expressed by the needs of the organization. . . ."[4]

Haimann suggests that an important function of human resource management is that of influencing. He states that the "influencing function is that function by which the supervisor evokes action from others to accomplish organizational objectives. It is the process that management uses to achieve goal-directed action from subordinates and colleagues."[5] In other words, the supervisor is a key to influencing employees to work productively.

Most successful businesses recognize that high productivity springs from a creative, innovative work environment. Most employees want to do a good job. The supervisor needs to understand that human behavior is based on the pursuit of unsatisfied needs and recognize that these needs vacillate within the individual's environment. The successful supervisor places emphasis on meeting the individual's needs as well as the organization's, and on the release of human potential.

Evaluating the situation

The humanistic approach encourages the supervisor faced with a difficult employee to evaluate the situation thoroughly and objectively be-

The humanistic approach encourages the supervisor faced with a difficult employee to evaluate the situation thoroughly and objectively before confronting the employee.

fore confronting the employee. There are several questions the supervisor might ask, such as the following.

1. Is the employee well informed? Was the employee communicated with prior to a change initiated by the supervisor? Are there weekly or monthly conferences just for communicating?
2. What is the degree of employee participation in your department? Do your employees set their own goals? Are there rewards for creative, innovative, highly productive employees?
3. Are the performance standards and expectations of employees realistic, clearly communicated and consistently interpreted? Are such standards and expectations discussed when the employees are hired? Are job expectations reviewed annually to make sure they are still meaningful, realistic and needed?
4. What procedures and techniques are used in hiring, placing and orienting employees? Does orientation include the overall organizational and departmental goals? What educational or training programs exist for your employees? Are they ongoing, planned at the level of needs of all employees and open to all levels of workers? Are employees involved in planning educational programs?
5. Are your employees dissatisfied with the work environment? If so, how are you responding?

These questions are not exhaustive, but they can stimulate the supervisor to evaluate his or her own style of managing human resources and to think of new approaches.

Taking disciplinary action

Supervisory reference materials, educational programs and personnel departments provide a major source of information on the tools and procedures for taking disciplinary action. One approach is the progressive disciplinary system where the supervisor (1) informally discusses problem behavior with the employee, (2) gives the employee an oral warning, (3) gives the employee a written warning, and (4) lays off or suspends, or demotes or discharges the employee. Some basic concepts to keep in mind when disciplining an employee are: always discipline in private; never lose your temper; direct your action against the act or behavior, not the person; and keep pertinent and accurate documentation of inappropriate behavior and disciplinary action.

When dealing with an employee who has exhibited inappropriate behavior, it is important to listen to the employee's side of the story. The supervisor should not assume that the employee has consciously set out to "do wrong" or "make life miserable," or that the employee "should know better," "doesn't care," "is lazy," etc. The supervisor should sensitively review the work environment and the employee's understanding of the job, work standards, expectations, procedures, etc. When the employee behaves inappropriately, the supervisor should speak with him or her after the behavior occurs. Why does the employee think he or she behaved that way? Does the employee see the behavior as being inappropriate or unacceptable?

It is usually best not to make any decisions about the employee's behavior at an initial conference. Rather, indicate to the employee your concerns and tell him or her that you will review all of the facts of the incident and that the two of you will meet again. Set a time and date to meet, preferably no longer than three to five days after the initial meeting.

The employee will likely feel that he or she is receiving fair treatment and that you have listened and will consider his or her side of the issue. If the behavior involves a serious offense or infraction against policy (e.g., theft, intoxication on duty or assault), the employee should be suspended immediately. Most personnel departments have clear directives and standard procedures for handling serious offenses. If the facts of a serious infraction prove the employee to be guilty, then the employee can be terminated at once. If the suspended employee is found not guilty, the suspension can be lifted and the employee reimbursed for the days of suspension. Suspension is an effective management tool since neither the organization nor the innocent employee lose in the long run.

Before deciding to take disciplinary action, the supervisor would do well to consider the following.

- Do I have a "square peg in a round hole"? Does the employee fit into the organization, the department, the job? Is there another job more suited to the employee's abilities?
- What are the performance standards for this job? Were they communicated to the employee? What does his or her record state about past performance? Can and should the performance standards be changed?
- What is the actual degree of difference between the employee's performance and what is desired or expected? Do the end results

and the employee's performance differ only on procedural points? If so, can the difference be tolerated, accepted or even adopted as a better way of doing the job?

- Should orientation and educational programs be strengthened?
- Am I thinking creatively, innovatively, humanistically? Or am I inflexible and securely tied to the way things have always been done?
- Is the employee's behavior really unacceptable in that it will diminish effectiveness and productivity and affect other workers or cause overall disorder in the desired state of affairs?
- Would I consider this unacceptable behavior from any employee under my supervision? Am I sure it is the behavior that I am reviewing and evaluating and not the person?
- What is my frame of mind concerning this employee? Is there a clash of values or personalities? Am I defensive about my authority, values and orders? Do I have a major concern about my boss

and his or her opinion of my supervision?

A supervisor who takes the time to evaluate an employee's behavior within the proper perspective of time, circumstances and frame of mind will often find a basically acceptable employee who simply needs some direction and a rechannelling of ability and energies. With such guidance, the employee may eventually become an asset to both the department and the organization.

MEETING THE CHALLENGE

Recognizing human needs and practicing the humanistic approach to managing human resources will prove highly productive. Supervisors will always have "difficult employees," but effective supervision can usually tap these people's potential, leading to happier employees and enhanced productivity. Often the difficult employee will provide the supervisor with a real challenge—a challenge for creativity, innovativeness and flexibility, and a challenge for growth and development for the department and employees.

REFERENCES

1. Bennett, A. *Improving Management Performance in Health Care Institutions* (Chicago: American Hospital Association 1978) p. 108.
2. Ibid. p. 109.
3. Haimann, T. *Supervisory Management for Health Care Institutions* (St. Louis, Mo.: Catholic Hospital Association 1973) p. 267–268.
4. Ibid. p. 268.
5. Ibid. p. 213.

Dealing with the angry employee

D. Douglas Dorman
Director of Personnel
Shenango Valley Osteopathic
*   Hospital*
Farrell, Pennsylvania

YOU ARE having a busy morning. Your department is going through another state inspection in two days and a visitor with an appointment is waiting to see you. Suddenly the administrator's secretary arrives with an employee, one of the people in your department who works nights, who is visibly upset. She explains, "Mr. Johnson wanted to see the administrator. When I explained that he was out of town, Mr. Johnson said he wanted to talk to someone right now. I brought him here because the assistant administrator won't be back until late this afternoon."

As a supervisor, how would you react? There are a number of things one could do under the circumstances, but the decision must be made quickly. An angry or upset employee can present fully as much of a crisis as equipment failure or a lack of supplies. A single mishandled incident

Health Care Superv, 1984,2(4),13–23
© 1984 Aspen Publishers, Inc.

can lead to lawsuits, union organizing activities, sabotage or deteriorating employee relations.

No supervisor likes to deal with an angry employee. Yet preparation for such an eventuality is an invaluable form of insurance.

THE INITIAL ENCOUNTER

The first few moments after you realize that an employee is angry are crucial in pointing the way toward satisfactory resolution of the problem. The first decisions to be made concern the time and the place to discuss the issue, not how to resolve the issue. The hallway and the cafeteria are places where such confrontations often begin and end, usually with both parties displeased with the results.

Place is the first priority. Even if you can spare only 60 seconds at that particular time, bring the person to an empty room where the two of you can talk in privacy. If the individual is on duty and cannot leave the work area, respect that necessity and agree on a time when the two of you can talk in private. Refuse to discuss a volatile issue with an employee in a non-private setting, making it clear that it is the time and place that cause your unwillingness to talk and not the subject at hand. The established time should be as soon as possible; anger can be like an untreated wound, festering and spreading. Recognizing there is a problem by agreeing to an early appointment is the first step toward defusing anger.

If the initial encounter occurs in "your territory" or if the employee has come to see you by appointment, again consider *place* first. If you have an office, close the door, turn off any music or other controllable distraction, sit down and give the employee your full attention. If your schedule is such that you cannot possibly engage in a long conversation just then, make it clear at the outset that you have only 5, 10 or 15 minutes you can spare. The employee may feel the issue can be resolved in that period of time, and may proceed. If not, agree on a time when a longer discussion can take place. If you do not have an office or are a long way from your normal work area, the two of you should agree on a time and place to talk further.

One other factor requires consideration. No schedule is so inflexible that it cannot be rearranged periodically. If the issue at hand is of greater importance than your scheduled meeting or appointment, decide to address it at that moment. Time is one of the most important resources you have to manage, and considering time to be flexible can help you concentrate your efforts on priority matters.

THE INTERVIEW: PHASE ONE

It is not usually difficult to begin talking with an angry employee. However, before allowing the employee to proceed, the manager has several responsibilities to meet. The setting, as noted, should be quiet, private and free from distractions. A time frame should be discussed, *if* time is going to be tight. For example, an explanation along the lines of "I have a meeting in half an hour, but we can continue our conversation later if we don't finish now." will allow you to end the conversation without offending the employee. Glancing frequently at your watch or trying to end an interview by hurrying through it can exacerbate the employee's anger.

The supervisor must remain aware of body language and use it to his or her advantage. Both manager and employee should be sitting, with eyes approximately on the same level. When one is sitting on a desk or counter and is looking down at the other, the person in the lower position may either feel intimidated and defensive or react as though being patronized. Chairs should be comfortable but not overstuffed or reclining. Enough "personal space" should be allowed between the chairs to allow both participants to feel at ease. Depending on circumstances, the manager may or may not want to sit behind a desk; this lends authority to the manager, but may inhibit the employee from expressing himself or herself as freely as might be the case in a more open seating arrangement.

Once both are seated, the manager should lean forward and initiate eye contact as he or she asks the employee to proceed. The employee should feel that he or she has the manager's undivided attention for as long as has been promised.

The manager should begin in a friendly tone even if the employee is hostile. The emphasis at the beginning should be to establish an atmosphere in which the employee can speak openly without fear of recrimination. A neutral inquiry works best, giving no opinion on the subject or second-guessing what the problem is. "You had something you wanted to discuss with me; go ahead," is usually enough to start the employee talking.

The emphasis at the beginning should be to establish an atmosphere in which the employee can speak openly without fear of recrimination.

The first part of the interview belongs to the employee. Unless asked a direct question, your *sole* responsibility is to listen actively to the entire message—the spoken words, the meanings "between the lines" and the body language.

A number of elements must be identified in the initial phase of the interview. These include what the problem is, how it developed and how and if the employee expects it to be resolved. The temptation to jump to conclusions or offer a "quick fix" must be avoided. Reflecting the employee's own thoughts and comments through such phrases as, "What I hear you saying is . . . ," or simply, "In other words . . . ," will allow the employee to continue the train of thought with the assurance that the message is getting across. "I can understand how you feel," is a phrase that comes readily to mind in meetings such as this, but it is one that can produce a great deal of resentment and should thus be avoided.

If the employee begins with a string of four-letter words or threatens to sue the institution, some intervention on the part of the manager is called for. Deflecting the anger away from you personally by asking the employee to be as specific as possible can help the individual focus on the particular problem causing the anger. If the person has trouble defining the problem, ask for the specifics of *what* or *at whom* he or she is angry. Following the response with "Why?" will often prompt a statement of the central issue from even the most laconic employee.

Questions are best left until the employee finishes the story. Interrupting, except to ask for clarification of a point that is preventing you from understanding the situation, can prevent the employee from presenting a cohesive narrative. Questions that are not directly related to the employee's concerns give the impression that the concerns are not being heard; by leaving questions to the end, you will be more aware of what those concerns are and can ask questions that are more pertinent to the situation. Let the employee do the talking; sometimes having a willing listener and a chance to talk through a problem out loud are all that are required.

There is one important exception to the foregoing advice: You should interrupt firmly if the employee remains angry but refuses to identify a particular issue or problem. If the person continues in that manner, explain that if the meeting proceeds in the present tone the session will be unproductive and the employee will be no better off for having talked. Reschedule the appointment, if necessary, and do not get drawn into the employee's emotional turmoil by responding with your own anger and frustration.

Keys to Effective Handling of an Angry Employee

1. Discuss the issue in private.
2. Allow adequate time for discussion.
3. Listen to what the employee says:
   A. What is the problem?
   B. How did it occur?
   C. What does the employee expect?
4. Grant the request, if reasonable.
5. Get all the facts you need.
   A. Interview other personnel.
   B. Review any documentation.
6. Use all your resources to develop a mutually satisfactory solution.
7. If a desired solution cannot be offered, explain why not.
8. Stay calm!

THE INTERVIEW: PHASE TWO

Once the employee has finished his or her story, you should have identified the problem, how it arose and how the employee expects it to be resolved. If these elements have not yet been identified, the first questions from the manager should be directed toward obtaining this vital information. Too often, managers expend needless energy trying to solve a problem that is not really an issue, or for which the employee has already determined a reasonable solution. Both the problem and the proposed solution should be paraphrased aloud by the manager so that both parties are sure to be working on the same problem. Failure to confirm the problem issue can result in misunderstandings that negate the efforts of both manager and employee.

After you have heard the employee's story and have obtained specific information, ask yourself whether the employee's request for action is reasonable. If the request can be granted without injuring others or expending a great deal of resources, grant the request. A quick response to a reasonable request can generate good will and establish your credibility as a manager who both listens to and cares about the employees. Unfortunately, however, the fact that the employee has reached the stage of anger probably indicates that he or she has already encountered obstacles to the desired goal. These must also be identified, together with any other issues that have not yet been taken into consideration, but that, nonetheless, must be seen as factors important in resolving the problem. What the employee is seeking may, for example, work well in your department, but it may cause problems in another department. If so, the manager must bring such other factors to the attention of the employee and seek to ar-

rive at a solution satisfactory to all parties.

If granting the request is not a simple task, the basic elements that you learned from the employee's story are where you should begin working on the problem. Knowing how the problem arose can sometimes allow a logical retracing of steps that will alleviate the situation. A new policy, for example, may have resulted in undue hardship for an employee due to circumstances no one who was involved in drafting the policy could have foreseen. The question to ask yourself is, "Is what happened to this employee fair and was it the expected result of our actions (in this case, the intention of the policy)?" Policies are not written in stone, and modifying or even retracting an ill-considered policy may be the solution. Similarly, other decisions made by a manager should be reexamined as to their merits. The manager who is willing to admit he or she has made a mistake will find that employees are less defensive when they themselves have made a mistake.

Often an employee's anger is directed at a particular individual who the employee feels has wronged him or her. Again, the role of the active listener is crucial to the manager seeking to resolve the situation amicably. The supervisor should not pass judgment on another employee in the presence of the angry employee; taking sides before hearing all aspects of a story amounts to assuming a conclusion without having all the facts. Committing yourself to supporting the employee's stance without getting the other party's opinions and, ideally, those of an independent party, can result not only in further complications of the issue but also in damage to your overall credibility as a fair and impartial arbiter.

If the anger is directed at another employee, it will be virtually impossible to resolve the situation in the first meeting. What you must decide is whether the next step in the process is a face-to-face meeting between the two parties with a third party (you) present or a private meeting between you and the individual at whom the employee's complaint is directed. In most cases, the latter course is preferable because the individual at whom the anger is directed should be given a chance to speak without the angry employee providing an intimidating or upsetting presence. If the stories conflict, a meeting of all three is then appropriate. You should present a synopsis of each of the two stories, explaining where the conflicts in the two views lie. Ask both parties if you presented their sides fairly and ask if there is some way to corroborate the parts of the stories that conflict. If the situation results in a stalemate—if both parties maintain their accounts of what happened—indicate that the situation will be documented, with both parties' input recorded, and that any future occurrences of similar situations should be reported to you at once. The important matter on which to focus at this time is preventing future

problems of a similar type, not ascertaining who is to blame for the current conflict. Even if a party is identified as being at fault in a given situation, the focus should remain on the future and how to keep as many people as possible (not just the angry employee) satisfied. If there is a "guilty" party, and there has been an incident that must be pursued through disciplinary channels, such action should take place between the manager and the offender and *not* in the presence of the employee who called the matter to your attention (albeit in an angry fashion).

There are occasions when a meeting of all three parties is appropriate without first holding an interview with the individual at whom the employee's anger is directed. If the anger is the direct result of something for which the other person is not directly responsible (for example, for following a specific policy or procedure), that individual may be brought into the session to discuss what happened. If the angry employee begins to direct inappropriate comments to the other person, your role is to keep the discussion focused on three key elements: what happened, why it happened and what can be done to correct the problem. Allowing employees to focus on personality conflicts is both nonproductive and demoralizing. As in the individual employee interview, you should refuse to continue a meeting in which either of the two parties will not discuss the issues in a calm and rational manner.

Allowing employees to focus on personality conflicts is both nonproductive and demoralizing.

When the employee is angry at another person, you need to consider the working relationship between the parties. The person at whom the anger is directed may be the angry employee's peer, supervisor or subordinate; he or she may be in another department, not at all affecting the employee according to the organizational chart, or the person may be one of many outside parties ranging from auditors to deliverers who influence the work of employees. Once the person at whom the anger is directed has been identified, a logical plan of action can be developed. The initial interviews are always necessary to determine the facts of the situation, but how to proceed once those facts have been obtained will depend on the organizational relationship between the parties to the conflict.

THE NEXT STEP: CONFLICT RESOLUTION

Once the nature of the problem is clear, and assuming that resolution did not result from the face-to-face meeting between the parties involved, organizational factors must be taken into account. In some cases, not even the fact-finding interviews can take place without consulting the appropriate department heads to allow the individuals involved to dis-

cuss the situation. Once the facts are available, the affected supervisors and managers should be made aware of the situation unless the employee has requested that the situation be held in confidence.

Confidentiality often presents a fine line for the manager to walk. Agreeing to hold personal or private information in confidence certainly is appropriate, but the manager should make clear that his or her first loyalty must remain with the institution. With such an understanding in place, the employee will have to decide exactly what to share; no false expectations will have been created. As with other confidential matters, the situation should not be discussed with persons who are not affected by it.

If the conflict lies with a co-worker of the angry employee, both parties will be under your supervision, so it is your responsibility to resolve the situation. However, this does not mean that you are entirely on your own or that you must come up with all the right answers at the time you are interviewing the employees involved. Once you have the facts, you can promise an answer by a specific date, not too far in the future but far enough ahead to give you time to reflect in peace and also to consult others who are either involved or who may have experienced a similar situation. Resources are available to you; do not try to resolve every conflict on your own, particularly if the issue lies outside your area of expertise. *Your* supervisor may provide insight by virtue of his or her experience. Your personnel director has undoubtedly handled any number of employee conflicts and can bring another perspective to the situation. Your peers at other institutions whom you have met at professional meetings may well have experienced similar conflicts. All these resources should be kept in mind and used as needed. No one can reasonably expect you to have all the answers, but as an effective manager, you had best know where to begin to look for them. There is no shame in seeking help and weighing advice; a problem only gets worse when it is ignored simply because you cannot think of a satisfactory solution.

If the angry employee is a supervisor who is upset with a subordinate, that supervisor should, like any other angry employee, be allowed to tell his or her complete story without interruption. Usually such a supervisor is only looking for a chance to blow off steam or to confirm a plan of action already thought through. On the other hand, a supervisor angry at a subordinate and unable to suggest a plan to resolve the conflict may be having trouble managing his or her area of responsibility. The anger, and not the actual cause of the problem, should lead you to counsel the supervisor; a supervisor who cannot resolve a conflict with a subordinate may be in need of additional management training. No supervisor is required to like all employees, but must nevertheless be able to work well with them—an impossible task if the supervisor remains angry at one or more of the employees.

Often an angry employee will be upset with his or her immediate supervisor, which, possibly, may be you. Again, the key is to focus on the source of the anger—the particular action or set of circumstances that resulted in the situation. One common source of such anger lies in unsatisfactory performance evaluations. An employee may feel that he or she has been rated unfairly, while the supervisor may consider the appraisal objective and accurate. It may seem as though there is no middle ground, but there are always alternatives to the seemingly typical win-or-lose conflict. The evaluation should be reviewed and discussed point by point, making changes where both parties feel it is appropriate. The employee, if still not satisfied, should be given the opportunity to respond to the evaluation in writing, with the assurance that the response will be placed in the employee's personnel file along with the evaluation itself. (Evaluations should not be sent out of the institution, and the entire contents of the personnel file should be taken into consideration when completing reference requests or when reviewing the person for possible promotion.)

When the conflict occurs between one of your employees and a person outside your department, the chain of command must be observed. As a supervisor, you cannot automatically "supervise" any nonmanagerial employee. That employee's supervisor will have to be advised of the situation and be given as many facts as you have available. The resolution of the conflict will most likely involve the participation of both supervisors. Implementation of a solution will proceed best if both supervisors have had a chance to address the issues they consider important and both have helped derive the plan of action. Even if the action to be taken is the same as the original supervisor would have suggested, the additional communication will improve the chances for successful implementation.

Conflict may sometimes occur between an employee and an individual not employed by the institution. This may involve a patient, a salesperson, a contractor or a physician, among others. While each of these categories must be handled somewhat differently, there are common principles among them. Determining the facts remains the first step, with the inclusion of the second party depending on circumstances. If, for example, a nurse complains that a particular patient is making lewd remarks to the nurses, such a complaint may be readily verified without interviewing the patient. Resolution may involve talking with the patient, but the decision to ask the patient to stop the lewd remarks can be decided on without a meeting between the patient and the complaining nurse and without interviewing the patient first. An accusatory approach would not be appropriate, because the patient may see as simple fun what the nurse finds offensive.

Conflicts with physicians fall into a special category because of the unique relationship between the physician and the hospital. The department manager generally has no authority over a staff physician and involving the chief of staff should usually be considered only as a last resort. Once the employee has made clear why he or she is angry with a particular physician, several courses of action are available. The employee may be satisfied with documentation of a particular incident, with further action occurring only when and if similar acts occur. The employee may have taken offense at a particular remark that was delivered offhand and was not meant to be taken seriously. Pointing out such a context may alleviate the situation. On the other hand, a physician who continuously offends employees by treating them as inferior, by making sexually harassing remarks or by otherwise upsetting staff through inappropriate behavior, must be addressed. The culture of the particular institution, as well as the personality of the particular physician, must be taken into account in determining how to proceed. The administrator may need to become involved as the only employee to discuss the situation with the physician. In other situations, such as one in which the manager knows the physician well, the manager may wish to discuss the matter with the physician personally and in private.

The employee who was angry should not be involved in this interview, as the physician may feel a need to "save face" and be unwilling to speak openly in front of the employee.

WHEN THE EMPLOYEE IS AT FAULT

Discussion has thus far focused on ways to handle an angry employee who has a legitimate complaint. However, the most difficult type of angry employee to face is the employee who holds unrealistic expectations about a given situation. For example, an employee who has worked eight hours of overtime each week for the last three months may feel that the overtime represents money he or she has the right to count on. The sudden addition of new staff to cover those hours at straight time may be a perceived incursion into the employee's rights. Under such circumstances the anger may be no less real, but the legitimacy of the rationale to hire new staff is unquestionable. The employee should, as always, be given the chance to express his or her feelings. The manager must then explain the rationale behind the decision, trying to make the employee understand why the decision was the best for the institution. It would be naive to expect every employee to come away satisfied from such a conversation, but at least the time will have been taken to explain *why* the decision that offended the employee was not arbitrary.

Sometimes a necessary management decision has unforeseen ramifications, but the decision is for some reason irrevocable. The angry employee, when he or she has explained the source of anger, should be told why the decision was made. The manager should take the time to explore different avenues of implementing the decision or of alleviating the hardships it may have caused this particular employee and other affected employees. Management is no less an art than a science, and creative answers to new problems should always be considered. Results count,

---

Management is no less an art than a science, and creative answers to new problems should always be considered.

---

and using all the resources available to you can make the desired results easier to obtain.

There will be circumstances under which the rationale for a particular decision cannot be revealed. It is better to say straightforwardly that there are aspects of the decision that you cannot discuss at this time, rather than to try to make up an answer. Once you have been trapped by a fabrication or an inconsistency, your word will count for little the next time a decision is challenged or a set of circumstances is questioned. Most employees can accept the fact that parts of your job cannot be discussed. As long as the reason you hold something in confidence is not just avoidance of discussion, refusing to discuss the matter is usually safe. Giving a limited amount of information or speaking in general terms is preferable to not discussing the situation at all. As in telling the truth, if your reason for holding something in confidence is only to avoid discussing an unpleasant topic, the long-range negative effects can easily outweigh the short-range benefits. If timing is critical, set a date when the issue can be discussed more freely. Health care institutions generally have well-developed grapevines, and what may seem like a wise decision to refuse to discuss a matter solely because of its volatility may backfire into concerted activity by a number of employees once the true circumstances come to light.

Finally, accept that you will not always be able to appease the angry employee. Unrealistic expectations or failure to grasp the "big picture" can result in a closed mind, an unwillingness to accept any decision other than what is already, to the employee, the right course of action. Once all of the possible explaining has been done, if the employee remains unhappy and dissatisfied the employee's further options may be outlined. The employee must either live with circumstances as they are, pursue the matter further through the chain of command or resign. While these options may seem limited and difficult to set forth, the employee must be made to realize that the institution must function at its best and can do so only when its employees work together whether or not they all agree with every action that occurs or every decision that is made.

POINTS TO REMEMBER

The supervisor will never enjoy a confrontation with an angry employee, but being prepared to handle such a situation in a systematic manner can make the experience less painful. Also, there are rewards to be earned in such situations, as when, for example, an employee enters your office angry but leaves satisfied that he or she has been heard and that the problem has been considered important enough to warrant some change. Even when you are unable to concede to the employee's desires, you can still perform a vital function—listening. As thoughtful managers are continually rediscovering, sympathetic listeners can go a long way toward dissolving anger.

Dealing with people who fail to produce

William Umiker
Adjunct Clinical Professor of Pathology
Pennsylvania State University
Hershey, Pennsylvania

PEOPLE WHO FAIL to produce can sap your energy and take a lion's share of your time. If you find yourself complaining about doing your work and theirs as well, it is time you did something about it. This article describes several such people and proposes suggestions for dealing with them.

The major categories of people who fail to produce are

- underperformers who can do no better,
- uninterested employees,
- people who work in spurts,
- passed-over employees,
- parents of latchkey children,
- people with personal problems,
- overstressed employees, and
- burnout victims.

UNDERPERFORMERS WHO CAN DO NO BETTER

These people lack both the necessary expertise and aptitude for the job. They

Health Care Superv 1989, 8(1), 68–74
©1989 Aspen Publishers, Inc.

should never have been hired in the first place. Try hard to identify such employees before the probationary phase is completed. Be prepared to justify your decision in case the person complains to the human resources department or levels charges of discrimination.

UNINTERESTED EMPLOYEES

Underperformance is often attributed to a poor attitude or a weak work ethic. The real reason may be boredom or dissatisfaction with the job, the work environment, or the other workers. Older workers who are just putting in time before retirement or who now work with much younger teammates are prime examples. There are often some employees who regard the job only as interim employment. People who have reached plateaus and people in dead-end jobs must also be included.

Learn the motivational needs of these people. Get them to see their opportunities to build on individual strengths and to use these strengths to grow. Consider the possibilities of job enrichment, cross-training, job rotation, special assignments, teaching responsibilities, or participation in some practical research projects. Provide more autonomy so that they feel in charge of their work. Workers' motivation stems largely from being able to use their talents in their job.

Older employees may be motivated by assigning trainees to them. Take advantage of their experience and know-how. But be careful to limit the assignment to teaching tasks; you do not want negative attitudes rubbing off on new employees. Providing additional training or sending uninterested employees to professional meetings or workshops may also be effective.

Ensure that social needs are met. Do they prefer solo or group work? How do they get along with teammates? Consider transfer to a faster moving group, if practical.

Are their ego needs fulfilled? Do they get the attention and respect they think they merit? Make a special effort to promote their self-esteem. A job title change, one's own desk or nameplate, and increased responsibility or authority may make a big difference. Ask for their advice, and thank them for it. Improve interpersonal communication and understanding. Show more interest in their outside activities and families. In other words, get to know them better. A caveat is in order: Do not make promises of promotion when few or no such opportunities exist.

PEOPLE WHO WORK IN SPURTS

In most departments there is at least one person who outperforms the others when he or she gets with it. The trouble is that these people work in spurts. In between bursts of energy they waste time gabbing or doing personal chores such as making up meal lists or balancing checkbooks. When you complain, they challenge you to prove that they are not doing as much or more than others.

Try assigning these hot-and-cold performers additional and more challenging assignments. If they balk, tell them that their periods of inactivity have a detrimental effect on the morale of their associates. One of the best solutions is to combine a spurt worker's job with that of a departing employee and attach a hefty pay raise to the resulting new position.

PASSED-OVER EMPLOYEES

Sally lost out on a promotion. Now she is less productive and vocally critical. Her former teammate, Sue, who was promoted, now must deal with Sally.

Sue can try to get Sally to serve as her advisor and backup. She could give Sally some choice assignments and delegate some administrative responsibilities to her. If Sally remains resentful and obstructive, Sue must have a frank dialogue with her, stating exactly what she will not tolerate and what she expects.

PARENTS OF LATCHKEY CHILDREN

Parents of children who return from school to empty homes are understandably concerned about the welfare of their off-spring. This results in telephone calls and mental distractions that can interfere with work performance.

Most of us are not qualified to counsel people about financial, emotional, or substance abuse problems, but we should be able to discern how these problems affect work.

Show these parents how their work is affected and ask how you can help. Sometimes the child can go to the home of a classmate or a relative. Suggest that the telephone calls be made during breaks.

Request that the calls be limited to a certain length.

Assign low priority tasks to the time of day when the greatest concern exists. Be tolerant about permitting them to take off time when crises develop, but know where to draw the line.

PEOPLE WITH PERSONAL PROBLEMS

Valuable employees sometimes go through trying periods because of family or financial difficulties. Over the short haul, be compassionate and understanding. Tell them you realize what they are going through and ask how you can help. Maybe their work hours can be modified, or special leave can be granted. Perhaps they could be relieved of certain responsibilities for a time. However, if this drags on and work really suffers or their associates grow restless, these people may have to be replaced.

Most of us are not qualified to counsel people about financial, emotional, or substance abuse problems, but we should be able to discern how these problems affect work. It is our responsibility to take action. To avoid legal traps or violating confidentiality or making matters worse, stick strictly to performance deficiencies and do not try to diagnose and treat the underlying cause.

Your goal is to get the employee to realize that his or her job is in jeopardy and to seek professional help. Most organizations have employee assistance programs (EAPs) for that purpose. Consult with your local EAP specialist when you think you have an employee with such a problem.

Suspect a personal problem when you observe increased absenteeism, frequent absence from the work area, confusion or difficulty in concentrating, reduced productivity or diminished work quality, friction with other employees, unusual behavior such as temper tantrums or social withdrawal, or proneness to accidents. Suspect drug problems when, in addition to the above, you notice that an employee meets with strangers or employees from other departments in the parking lot, is suspected of theft, makes secretive telephone calls, stays in the washroom for long periods of time, wears dark glasses indoors, wears long-sleeved shirts in hot weather or has blood stains on sleeves, or perspires excessively.

In dealing with personal problems, document how performance or behavior has changed. You may need this document for subsequent administrative or legal action.

Hold a frank and firm counseling session. Describe the unsatisfactory work, not what you suspect to be the problem. Never voice suspicions of drug, alcohol, or psychiatric disorder. For example, say, "Jim, I am concerned about the number of errors I'm finding in.... Is something bothering you?" Do not say, "Jim you have a booze problem. You often have alcohol on your breath."

Listen attentively. If no explanation is offered, say, "I don't know what the problem is, and it's really none of my business, but your performance is my business. Something has to be done."

If performance fails to improve, repeat the counseling session, honing in on the underlying problem without being accusatory. For example, say, "Jim, I feel that something is really bugging you. Frankly, your job is in jeopardy. I would like you to talk to Miss Evans in our human resource department. She may be able to help you. Would you like me to make an appointment for you?" (What drug and alcohol abusers fear most is loss of job, because it means loss of the means to support their habit.)

If the employee cooperates and gets treatment, continue your support by expecting occasional backsliding, giving positive strokes for good work, resisting the temptation to lighten the workload, and treating the person the way you treat other employees. Remember that a reasonable transition period may be required before performance reaches the desired level. If the employee refuses to seek help, or if rehabilitation fails, take the necessary disciplinary action.

It is important to know the policy of your organization, document performance, use only job performance to initiate disciplinary action, be tough, but do not take punitive action until counseling has been attempted, show concern for the person, counsel in private, and set clear expectations. Do not ignore or delay, apologize for discussing performance deficiencies, lecture, try to be a diagnostician or therapist, get involved in discussing personal problems in depth, or moralize (there should be no stigma attached to personal problems). In addition, do not transfer their work to others, do it for them, or buy their phony excuses. Most important, do not give them performance ratings they do not deserve. This can come back to haunt you.

OVERSTRESSED EMPLOYEES

Stress factors over which supervisors have some control appear in the box, "Stress Factors Supervisors Can Affect." Signs of excessive stress are listed in the box, "Signs of Excessive Stress." Supervisors should be

---

Stress Factors Supervisors Can Affect

- Poor general supervisory practices
- Too little or too much communication
- Time pressures and deadlines
- Lack of equipment or supplies
- Unclear or excessive performance expectations
- Too little or too much responsibility
- Lack of training for assigned tasks
- Territorial disputes
- Lack of performance feedback
- Oppressive, ambiguous, or unfairly enforced policies or rules
- Stifled creativity or career development
- Demands for perfection
- Working with difficult people

---

able to reduce the stress that they cause, institute measures to increase stress resistance in their teammates, recognize the signs of excessive stress, and take remedial measures to help a distressed person. In short, they should help people become resistant to stress.

There are three key factors in stress resistance: self-esteem, assertiveness, and con-

---

Signs of Excessive Stress

- Excessive sick leave, absenteeism, or tardiness
- Inability to get along with others
- Decreased work quality and productivity
- Increased use of tobacco, alcohol, or drugs
- Emotional outbursts
- High-pitched, nervous laughter
- Increased irritability
- Trembling, tics, or stuttering
- Complaints of: anxiety or depression; high blood pressure; duodenal ulcers; cardiac irregularities; chronic fatigue; insomnia, nightmares; headaches, backaches, or premenstrual tension; or loss of appetite or compulsive eating.

---

trol. These factors are closely interrelated. Assertiveness facilitates open, clear communication and promotes a feeling of being in control.

Several studies have shown the importance of being in control. In one example, assembly line workers were given permission to stop or change the speed of their production line, and morale, productivity, and work quality all increased.

Workshops and publications that teach assertiveness and stress management are available to almost everyone. Wise supervisors encourage their personnel to take advantage of these learning experiences. Schedule staff presentations on stress management. The importance of nutrition, exercise, and relaxation techniques can be reinforced.

People must have clear expectations and must be able to meet these expectations.

Building self-esteem is more complex. It demands good training, coaching, and supporting. Make certain that position descriptions are based on competency, indoctrination programs are thorough, and educational measures are based on needs assessment. People must have clear expectations and must be able to meet these expectations. Help each employee to become an expert in some aspect of his or her work. Being the most knowledgable person and being consulted are great for self-esteem. Make people feel needed. Acknowledge employee contributions at meetings, in newsletters, and in memorandums to higher authorities.

Provide frequent feedback on performance. Objective and empathetic performance reviews and planning sessions can help. Respond to boredom and frustration before they get out of control. Stress is much more likely to result from frustration than from overwork. Use counseling to help individuals who experience internal stressors such as ambition, competitiveness, or materialism or nonwork external stress elements related to social, family, or financial problems.

Several ways to reduce stress follow:
- Eliminate the stress factors listed in the box, "Stress Factors Supervisors Can Affect."
- Develop a fun ambience: Encourage humor and laughter.
- Do not overwhelm people with assignments for which they are not qualified.
- Reinforce good performance with praise. Be careful how you react to mistakes.
- Do not make major changes too suddenly or without preparing the people who are affected.
- Give people more leeway in how they get their job done.
- Do not assign highly stressful tasks to persons who have a low stress threshold.
- Reduce the workload of overachievers.
- Protect subordinates from the attacks of physicians and any others who tend to abuse them.

BURNOUT VICTIMS

Burnout is an advanced stage of overstress. Burnout victims have lost their coping ability. The overloading of job-related emotional circuits results in a feeling of

Signs of Burnout

- Depression
- Self-deprecating outlook
- Chronic fatigue
- Irritability
- Loss of enthusiasm
- Loss of idealism, energy, and purpose
- Cynicism and fault finding
- Anger addressed toward job, superiors, and peers
- Procrastination
- Resistance to change
- Withdrawal from fellow workers, or sometimes family and friends
- Lack of participation at meetings
- Talk of moving to a farm or distant place

powerlessness. In addition to emotional exhaustion, there is a shift toward negative attitudes and a sense of personal devaluation.

The burnout syndrome is characterized by exhaustion on all levels—physical, emotional, and attitudinal. The signs and symptoms are similar to those of overstress. The inability to cope is manifested by the signs listed in the box, "Signs of Burnout." The destruction of coping ability is often related to unattainable goals, absence of clear or desired outcomes, lack of recognition or feedback, feeling of powerlessness or lack of control, loss of self-esteem, or lack of assertiveness.

Pep talks are ineffective. Try to build a more supportive relationship. Here are some specific remedial measures:
- Institute antistress measures (see previous notes).
- Formulate clear-cut and attainable goals with the employee.
- Get the person to focus on one day at a time and not dwell on past or future concerns.

- Help the person to accept his or her limitations.
- Reassign the employee or change the work schedule.
- Recommend counseling.
- Consider a change of job or perhaps retirement.

•   •   •

There are many causes of underperformance. To achieve increased productivity without sacrificing work quality, an accurate diagnosis and appropriate remedial measures are necessary. This presentation provides practical clues for correctly diagnosing underperformance, and offers pragmatic approaches to its resolution.

Handling manipulation

Ruth Davidhizar
Director of Nursing
Logansport State Hospital
Logansport, Indiana

MANIPULATION IS the conscious or unconscious use of indirect means to achieve a goal.[1] While manipulation may be used in a positive way to meet personal and professional objectives, manipulation encountered by a nurse is often negative and even destructive.[2] Destructive manipulation is characterized by lack of consideration for others in order to meet one's own immediate wants and needs.

Nurses encounter manipulation in interactions with patients, patients' families, those they supervise, and others with whom they come in contact. If a nurse is unknowingly manipulated, feelings of powerlessness and distress may result and nursing goals may be thwarted. A nurse must be not only able to recognize manipulation, but also skilled in handling this powerful interpersonal phenomenon if effective work relationships are to be maintained. This article addresses this important issue by describing both manipulators and nurses susceptible to

Health Care Superv, 1990, 8(3), 37–44
© 1990 Aspen Publishers, Inc.

manipulation. Also, approaches are outlined for handling manipulation in others.

DYNAMICS OF DESTRUCTIVE MANIPULATION

Destructive manipulation serves to meet one person's needs at the expense of another; in other words, destructive manipulation exploits others. Techniques of destructive manipulation may range from wheeling and dealing to more passive and subtle maneuvering. Destructive manipulation often appears selfish, callous, irresponsible, and impulsive.[3] The manipulator who uses destructive techniques treats people as objects without consideration for self-esteem, interpersonal honesty, or closeness.[4] When people are treated as objects, they become dehumanized—mere tools to fulfill the manipulator's needs.[5]

Although manipulation is commonly considered to be negative, many manipulative techniques have no damaging effects and may even be constructive.[6] Manipulative techniques may achieve productive goals, satisfy the needs of everyone involved, and neither exploit nor take advantage of others. Some manipulative techniques may even boost morale, encourage productivity, and promote camaraderie. Constructive manipulation may be pleasurable not only to the manipulator, but also to the target. For example, a nurse who flatters a patient who successfully does an insulin injection for the first time or who commends a coworker for a contribution in a nursing meeting is manipulating, but may also be promoting positive feelings.

While little difficulty is encountered by the nurse when the manipulative interaction is pleasurable or productive, serious negative and destructive effects can occur when it is offensive. Manipulation that unfairly serves one's own purpose, clouds the real issues that need to be addressed, or creates discomfort or self-doubt requires intervention. However, before a nurse can handle manipulation, he or she must understand dynamics that operate in both manipulators and nurses susceptible to manipulation.

The manipulator

Manipulative behavior is often based in childhood experiences; a child may learn manipulative behavior by viewing it in others. For example, a child, viewing mother's pouting behavior as an effective control over father, may copy this behavior. A child may also use manipulation to attempt to gain control over the environment. For example, a child may cry in a store hoping to obtain a desired toy: If the crying is ineffective, the child may cry more loudly to gain attention from other customers or may try to induce guilt in the parent by saying, "You never buy me anything, but you always buy things for sister." Effective manipulative behavior may be learned as a child and used throughout life when control is desired. While some persons continue to use obvious forms of manipulation as adults, others learn more subtle manipulative techniques, which may be integrated with other, less objectionable interpersonal techniques and used with little objection from others.

Manipulative behavior is also rooted in an underlying fear and distrust of interpersonal honesty; a person may avoid truth and intimacy out of fear of being hurt. However, the desire for power and control and the desire for love and approval are strong, prompt manipulative interactions.[6] If manipulative behavior does not achieve the desired approval from others, feelings of insecurity may increase, and an individual may use manipulative behavior in increased efforts to relate to others.

A person who interacts in a manipulative way frequently lacks skill in more sophisticated interpersonal techniques. When initial manipulative techniques fail, other kinds of manipulative techniques, including the following, may be used.

Flattery

Some forms of flattery, charm, and compliment exploit the human desire to be needed and valued. When one person "butters up" another with an ulterior motive and lacks sincerity, the action can be considered a negative manipulative one. The following is an example: "You look so terrific today. That dress is so becoming! It makes your waistline look about 20. I really have been having trouble doing these care plans and you are so good at them. Do you think you could do this for me while I take my patient down to the beauty shop?"

Criticism

Criticism can also be used successfully as a manipulative technique to gain control over others. For example, a dietary employee may tell a nurse, "The nursing staff is so slow getting these meal trays out, it is no wonder the patients turn in all those complaints about the hospital." Since feelings of intimidation and anxiety are common responses to criticism, this comment may precipitate the behavior the critic desires.[7] Criticism may also prompt feelings of guilt and inadequacy, powerful weapons that can be used to persuade nurses to do what they do not wish to do or would not consider on their own.[8] For example, a quality assurance coordinator may say to a nurse, "This hospital will not get accredited if these care plans are not redone by the survey next week. I have not seen one decent care plan on this unit." This comment could create feelings of both guilt and inadequacy, and the nurse might redo the plans as a result.

Criticism can be given with the intent of causing discomfort. For example, one colleague may say to another, "You look a mess today. You must be having a hard time keeping up with your assignments. Maybe you need to request a transfer." This kind of a personal attack may be manipulative.

Other persons may feel attacked if they must wait for an appointment, if an interview is interrupted, or if they are treated as if they were ignorant. The manipulator may induce anxiety by refusing to listen, asking for statements to be repeated, or deliberately refusing eye contact in an interview.[9]

Criticism that is manipulative and may be destructive seeks to gain control of another's behavior through anxiety. This is in contrast to constructive criticism, which focuses on problematic behavior in a direct way and seeks to improve it through logical collaborative problem solving.

Calculated delay

Calculated delays, such as waiting until the last minute to make a decision, can induce psychological pressure and be a manipulative ploy. Creating the impression of a fading opportunity can also induce pressure and spur individuals to action. This comment is a good example: "This may be our last opportunity to make this change before we are surveyed. If we don't change now, we could lose our accreditation."

Complaints

Complaints are another type of destructive manipulation when they are used to motivate another to actions of rescue, as in the following case: "I always get the bad jobs around here. I'm tired of this. Why do I always get the dirty work?" Pointing out errors, deficiencies, or lack of experience can cause a nurse to feel insecure and thereby give another feelings of power. A patient may say, "You've never done this procedure before, have you? I want a nurse who really knows how to do it." With this comment, the patient may increase his or her own feeling of power by causing insecurity in the nurse.

Helplessness

Others may manipulate through helplessness and dependency. Nurses who do tasks others are "unable to do" or are "not good at" may be victims of manipulation: "You are so good at this and I'm so slow. Do you think you could take off this set of doctor's orders for me?" Crying, pouting, or "not talking" are other dependent manipulative techniques that may be used to gain control over others: "I'm so upset about my child being sick. I don't think I can get these medications out. Could you do it for me?"

Threats

Threats can also be a form of destructive manipulation. An individual who aligns with a group seen as powerful (e.g., the press, the union, the administration, or the physician) is often attempting to gain control by name-dropping. For example, a nurse may tell a nursing director, "I'll take this to

> *Some people have personal qualities, such as insecurity and fearfulness, that make them more susceptible and better targets for a manipulator.*

the union if you don't get me that vacation I requested. You are not being fair. You got the vacation you wanted. Why should the nurse managers get their vacation request, but not the nurses?" When threats are used, destructive manipulation may sound like blackmail: "If you report me for this, I'll tell the administration about certain things going on in the nursing department that would be very interesting to them."

A person attempting to negotiate may use threats to gain power in an interaction. A threat is easy to make; however, threats manipulate through pressure and may prove destructive to a relationship by making negotiation more difficult. For threats to be effective, they must be credibly communicated. A threat that lacks credibility will not manipulate; there must be a clear indication that the threat will and can be followed through.

Aggressive behavior

Aggressive behaviors such as sexual comments, touching, or aggressive questioning about personal matters may be used to create discomfort and self-doubt to gain power in an interaction. Additional methods of creating discomfort and self-doubt are domineering comments that exaggerate one's authority, strength, and power, such as: "I have been here a lot longer than you and I know what will work in this institution and with the employees. You don't have enough experience to know what will work here, even if you do have a degree."

Physical complaints

When physical complaints are used in an underhanded way to gain control over others, destructive manipulation may be present. Two examples follow: "I've got a sore throat, and I really can't do justice to that speech to the new volunteers today. You'll have to do it for me. We do want them to get a good impression of the hospital." Or, "I don't feel well, could you clean up the treatment room for me? I need to go lie down."

The person susceptible to manipulation

Since manipulation is an interpersonal process, it cannot occur if the person being manipulated is not susceptible to manipulation. Some people have personal qualities, such as insecurity and fearfulness, that make them more susceptible and better targets for a manipulator. Other personal qualities that may indicate vulnerability are a sense of obligation and responsibility, feelings of guilt, and a highly vulnerable appearance.

Insecurity and fearfulness

Personal and professional insecurity and fear often make a nurse susceptible to manipulation in the work environment. For example, a nurse who feels insecure about being replaced may agree to take on extra tasks, or may be more susceptible to a colleague's flattery as recognition of personal success. A nurse who is hesitant to offend others may hesitate to state personal opinions when asked.[8] A nurse who is insecure frequently has a strong desire to please

others, and is thus more vulnerable to manipulation.

A nurse who regards others with fear is also vulnerable to manipulation in the workplace. One who fears that love and approval will be withdrawn may comply with unreasonable demands. A nurse who fears what people will think may hesitate to take risks or to speak out in a group.

Sense of obligation or responsibility

A sense of obligation or duty places individuals in positions where they may feel vulnerable to manipulation. For example, a nurse may feel obligated to respond to patient complaints or to do everything he or she is directed to do in the workplace.

As professional helpers, nurses often feel responsible for handling needs that arise in the health care setting. Trained to be able to answer health questions, give care, and provide assistance, the nurse may feel obligated to step in and take over for someone who presents a complaint and appears in distress. Many nurses feel the need to rescue others in distress and are highly vulnerable to complaints of pain, requests for help, the appearance of helplessness, and other indications of trouble. Even when others are capable of assuming responsibility and need to do so in order to gain independent functioning, nurses often feel the urge to rush in to help the individual face a dilemma.

Guilt

Feelings of guilt may persuade nurses to behave in ways they would not otherwise consider. A nurse who feels guilty will be more easily manipulated. He or she may think, "I am being paid more than the aide, and it isn't fair that the least-paid staff have to do all the unpleasant jobs. She said she was busy. I can make some beds today." Or, "The patient hasn't been out of his room for week. I guess I can take him down the hall for a quick walk without a doctor's order. He can't help it if the doctor didn't write the order and I didn't remember to ask."

Appearance of vulnerability

Some nurses may be seen by others as more likely to be vulnerable to manipulative tactics. A nurse who is new on the job, who is carrying out an assignment for the first time, or who is seen as weak or timid may be a more likely target of manipulative efforts, since he or she may be seen as vulnerable.

Body language also may create an appearance of vulnerability to manipulation. A petite and quiet woman may be more likely to be the victim of a manipulator than a woman with a large frame and a loud voice. A person who sounds and appears assertive will be seen as less likely to respond to manipulative tactics and is thus less likely to be a target for manipulative behavior.

APPROACHES TO HANDLING MANIPULATION

A number of factors are involved in handling manipulative behavior in others. The nurse must be self-aware and alert for manipulative behavior in others. The dynamics behind the manipulative behavior should be assessed and responded to. Confrontation can assist manipulators to relate more directly, and limit-setting can increase both parties' feelings of security.

Self-awareness

The nurse's personal self-awareness is crucial to effectively handling manipulative

behavior. Nurses who are inexperienced or gullible should be careful to investigate situations adequately before taking action. Being too trusting can cause a nurse to be easily taken in. The nurse must be aware of personal feelings of insecurity, fear, responsibility, obligation, and guilt that increase susceptibility to manipulation. A nurse who is aware of presenting the appearance of vulnerability may choose to use more assertive body language and behavior in order to create a less vulnerable impression.

Alertness for manipulative behavior

The nurse should be alert for personal reactions that may indicate that manipulation is occurring. Feelings of powerlessness and of being used are common indications that manipulation is present in an interaction.[6] Feelings of anger and resentment directed at either the self or others may also be clues that manipulation is occurring. A nurse who understands the feelings precipitated by manipulative behavior can use this understanding to recognize subtle manipulation.

The dynamics behind manipulative behavior

Recognizing the cause of manipulative behavior is essential to effective handling of it. While some manipulation is part of a lifelong style of relating learned in childhood, many attempts at manipulation are precipitated by situations in the present that are causing transitory feelings of insecurity and powerlessness. While a lifelong style of relating may not be changed, feelings in the present situation can often be altered. If the nurse can help the person who feels powerless to gain some feeling of control in the situation, manipulative behavior may be decreased. For example, in response to a patient's relative who is complaining to the nurse about incompetent care, the nurse might say, "I realize you are worried about what will happen with your relative. I know the doctor is making rounds in an hour. If you want to come back at that time I can arrange for the doctor to talk with you."

Recognizing the cause of manipulative behavior is essential to effective handling of it.

The issue of control is crucial in responding to the manipulator. Allowing the manipulator to assume control over areas he or she is able to control will promote feelings of power. The nurse must be comfortable with giving up control in order to promote growth on the part of the other person.[10]

In cases of situational stress, it is often inappropriate for the nurse to respond to the manipulative behavior itself; instead, the focus should be on the cause of the feelings of powerlessness. When persons who feel powerless are assisted to verbalize their feelings, anxiety may decrease. If an open and direct discussion can occur, the need for indirect and manipulative behavior may decrease and problem solving can commence.

Aggressive techniques for reacting to manipulative behavior have been suggested in some nursing literature. These include fogging, in which the nurse agrees with manipulative critical statements; negative assertion, in which the nurse openly admits negative things about self; and negative inquiry, in which further criticism is prompted.[7] These techniques are not recommended in cases of situational stress, since they do not respond to the underlying dynamics that precipitated the behavior.

Confrontation

Confrontation is a significant technique for facilitating self-growth, resolving conflict, and prompting problem solving.[11] Manipulation should be confronted when it involves behavior in others that requires discipline or that negatively affects the performance of the health care team. For example, a supervisor could tell a problem employee, "You have been late getting your care plans done every week this month. You need to get these done on time even if you are busy with other things and aren't feeling well. If you are late again, I'm going to take disciplinary action."

Confrontation should be direct and matter-of-fact rather than sarcastic or punitive. Limits should be precisely defined and consequences of nonadherence clearly identified.

The most difficult task in using confrontation is often determining whether or not confrontation is appropriate and will be useful. Because resolution of problems is usually an objective of confrontation, confrontation may be contraindicated if no options are available.

Limit-setting

Limit-setting is a necessary response to some manipulative behavior and can increase feelings of security. "I am not able to stay in your room and talk with you any longer even though I would like to. What I can do is stop by later this morning to check on you. If you need anything, you can turn on your light and someone will come in."

The way limits are set is important. Even though a nurse may be angry with manipulative behavior, care should be taken to set limits without involving personal emotions. "I" messages should be stated in a firm yet kind manner. If the nurse sounds indecisive, the result may be more manipulation and testing.

If the limits can be negotiated before they are set, this can respond to the underlying need for power in the manipulator who feels powerless. Negotiating compromises can increase the self-esteem and feelings of control of both parties. But if the nurse's integrity is at stake, a compromise should not occur. For example, if a patient asks for pain medication when none is ordered, the requested medication cannot be supplied. If the hospital indicates that nurses can give Tylenol, the nurse may negotiate with the patient about this.

Once limits have been set, a reaction such as anger, defiance, or further manipulation may occur. If reactions to the limit-setting are inappropriate, this too must be dealt with.[2] Manipulators often comply with specific limits and then display aggression in other more subtle ways. For example, instead of coming in late and stating it was because of illness, the employee may ask to leave early for a doctor's appointment. Limits serve to provide an immature individual with a feeling of security: When limits are tested and found to be enforced, this enforcement will provide an additional feeling of security.

• • •

Nurses will regularly encounter manipulation during the workday. Since manipulation involves an interpersonal process in which the nurse must participate, self-awareness is crucial to effective handling of this complex interpersonal phenomenon. The nurse must assess and respond to the dynamics present in a manipulative interaction. Finally, limit-setting may increase feelings of security in a person who feels powerless.

REFERENCES

1. Phelps, S., and Austin, N. *The Assertive Woman.* San Luis Obispo, Calif.: Impact Publishers, 1973.
2. Davidhizar, R. "Using Manipulation to Your Advantage." *Nursing Management,* to be published.
3. Shostrom, E. *Man, The Manipulator.* Nashville, Tenn.: Abingdon Press, 1967.
4. Chitty, K., and Maynard, C. "Managing Manipulation." *Journal of Psychosocial Nursing* 24, no. 6 (1988): 10.
5. Kumler, F.R. "An Interpersonal Interpretation of Manipulation." In *Some Clinical Approaches to Psychiatric Nursing,* edited by S. Burd and B. Marshall. New York: Macmillan, 1963.
6. Payne, B. "Managing the Manipulator in the OR." *AORN* 26, no. 5 (1977): 839–41.
7. Smith, M.J. *When I Say No I Feel Guilty.* New York: The Dial Press, 1975.
8. Stanhope, M., and Lancaster, J. *Community Health Nursing.* St. Louis: C.V. Mosby, 1984.
9. Fisher, R., and Ury, W. *Getting to Yes.* Boston: Houghton Mifflin, 1981.
10. Haber, J., Leach, A.M., and Schudy, S.M. *Comprehensive Psychiatric Nursing.* 2d ed. New York: McGraw-Hill, 1984.
11. Davidhizar, R., and Bowen, M. "Confrontation, An Underused Management Technique." *Health Care Supervisor* 7, no. 1 (1988): 29–34.

Responding to the codependent employee

Ruth Davidhizar, R.N., D.N.S., C.S.
Assistant Dean and Chairperson for
  Nursing
Bethel College
Mishawaka, Indiana

IN RECENT YEARS *codependency* has become a familiar term. However, in spite of its familiarity, codependency is not well understood, and this term is often used without a clear understanding of its meaning. Since the 1970s, *codependency* has been used to describe an unhealthy pattern of coping that developed in reaction to an alcoholic or chemically addicted family member.[1] Others thought of codependency as a disease exhibiting a recognizable pattern of characteristics. As a disease, codependency was considered capable of creating sufficient dysfunction to warrant a diagnosis of mixed personality disorder.[2] The theoretical framework used by family counselors in response to codependency has also differed, that is, ego psychology, family systems, behavioral, and interpersonal.[3-6] Nevertheless, in spite of various treatment approaches, there has been general agreement that codependency was a predictable phenomenon in the family of a chemically dependent person.

Health Care Superv, 1992, 10(4), 36–44
©1992 Aspen Publishers, Inc.

Today, the term codependency is still used in relation to persons who develop a set of physical and psychological symptoms as a result of interaction with a family member who has a substance addiction. However, in addition to a relationship to such a person, codependency is used in a much broader way to describe an intrapsychic and interpersonal phenomenon that may occur in relationships in which dependency and control are issues.[7] Thus persons who let the behavior of others affect them or who are obsessed with controlling the behavior of others may be considered codependent.

Since codependent persons may be nurses, it is important for the nurse manager to understand both the development and characteristics of this phenomenon in order to respond appropriately. Productivity and morale improve if managers can control and even reverse codependent behavior of staff.

DEVELOPMENT OF CODEPENDENCY

The person who can be described as codependent exhibits a restricted pattern of coping with life that has developed out of prolonged exposure to a set of rules prohibiting open expression of feelings and direct discussion of problems.[8-10] While codependency often has its developmental roots in childhood, codependency is not an inherited behavior. Rather, individuals learn codependency in the context of relationships in which they believe they must assume responsibility (see box). Consider a child who assumes responsibility for cleaning, cooking, doing laundry, and caring for other siblings while mother is drunk and father is working.[10] While outwardly the image of strength and security is projected, a

---

Development of Codependency

1. Rigid situation in which child felt responsible for factors beyond personal control and could not express feelings about the role assumed
2. Lack of self-worth when control could not be gained over situation
3. Dependence on others for self-worth
4. Seeks situations in which others can be controlled, for example, employment in nursing and social service

---

codependent child inwardly feels insecurity, self-doubt, and confusion. Low self-esteem is at the core of the etiology of codependency. Self disparaging comments are commonly heard from the individual who is codependent: "Nobody asks my opinion," "Nobody cares what I think," or "I work harder than anybody and nobody appreciates it." In fact, Wegscheider-Cruse describes the codependent person as an individual who has failed to develop personal identity and "essence self-worth."[11]

It would appear that the need to be needed has prompted some individuals with codependency to enter professions that involve a "helping" role, such as nursing, social services, or the ministry. Codependency can prompt individuals to remain in an unhealthy and self-sacrificing relationship with an irresponsible person who has repeatedly let them down.

Recent estimates suggest that at least 28 million Americans or one out of ten individuals has grown up in a family conducive to developing characteristics of codependency in children.[8] Others say that number could easily be only a fraction of codependents. Because of the likelihood that codependents are attracted to the helping professions, it is especially significant for the health care manager to be cognizant of this pattern.

CHARACTERISTICS OF CODEPENDENCY

Codependency is characterized by excessive focus or dependency on relationships to others.[12] The codependent person is unusually concerned with what others think. The concern for what others think results in behavior that demonstrates excessive feelings of responsibility in personal and work relationships. There is excessive dedication to a cause. However, such overfunctioning often results in feelings of resentment later for having "rescued" others. Other features of codependency include the tendency to feel guilty when the perceived expectations of others are not fulfilled. Codependent individuals think they should be able to make those around them happy, and when this does not occur they feel they are inadequate.[13] Finally, in codependent individuals normal human feelings such as shame, fear, pain, and anger are so magnified that an emotional state marked by anxiety and irrationality is almost always present.

The over concern for others often triggers anger from those who are "cared for," in turn precipitating even more feelings of frustration, powerlessness, and poor self-esteem on the part of the codependent. This unrewarding cycle of events often leaves the codependent individual feeling mistrustful and insecure in relationships (see Figure 1). Since early childhood experiences have resulted in a significant lack of self-worth, the codependent person desires self-worth from other people. This process is described as "external referenting."[7(p.9)] In other words, if

children, spouse, parents, coworkers, or employers are happy, the codependent individual is happy; if they are sad, the codependent individual is sad.[7] Personal behavior is judged on the feedback obtained from others. Thus, approval from others is frequently solicited: "What do you think of how this turned out?" On the other hand, the codependent individual also assumes responsibility for the feelings and behaviors of others and consequently if they are unhappy,

---

Since early childhood experiences have resulted in a significant lack of self-worth, the codependent person desires self-worth from other people.

---

the codependent person feels personally at fault: "If I'd have gotten to work earlier this wouldn't have happened." The codependent person is fearful of being hurt or rejected by others and is highly sensitive to feelings and actions of others: "I didn't take that phone call. I wasn't even here. You can't blame me." Most importantly, the codependent person needs to feel needed in order to have a relationship.

The following specific behaviors may indicate the presence of codependency:

- dependency on others for approval,
- need to control people and situations,
- rigidity and perfectionism,
- difficulty adjusting to change,
- an excessive need to take care of others,
- feelings of powerlessness,
- feelings of low self-esteem and shame,
- difficulty in making decisions,
- feeling overresponsible for others,
- difficulty forming close relationships, and
- difficulty expressing feelings.

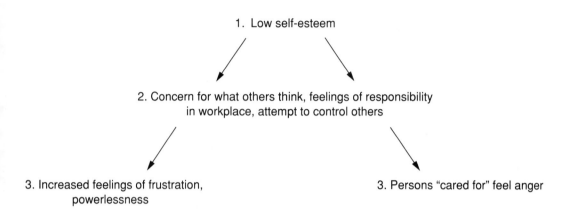

Figure 1. The cycle of codependence.

When the behavior of the codependent individual is identified as a problem in the workplace it is not because of quality or quantity of work. Rather the concern is for side issues that overshadow overall performance.[8(p.37)] For example, a codependent nurse may exhibit any of the following behaviors:

- repeatedly takes on heavier work assignments and more responsibility than assigned,
- has difficulty delegating work to others,
- often listens to difficulties of coworkers,
- has difficulty adjusting to changes in policies and procedures even when the changes will make the work easier,
- is frequently found in the middle of disputes between fellow employees,
- frequently complains about being overworked and underappreciated,
- evidences hypersensitivity to criticism about work especially when given by the supervisor,
- is loyal to others even when the performance of others is obviously poor,
- wants to be in control or avoids responsible positions, and

- worries how others will react to personal actions.

Codependency traits are not necessarily bad traits. In fact, most individuals have some tendency to codependency. Persons may possess situational codependency; for example, they may evidence dependency and anxiety after being told of poor performance but not demonstrate codependency as a personality style. Codependent behaviors may also be apparent around certain individuals but not around others; for example, an individual is codependent in a relationship with the supervisor but not with anyone else. The nurse manager should be alert for codependency both as a situational behavior and as a pervasive personality style. While a situational reaction may not require intervention, the manager's action may be necessary when a pervasive style is apparent (see Appendix).

Codependents often have a history of dependency on substances such as food, drugs, or alcohol. Unresolved codependency frequently results in the person switching to another compulsive behavior when a change in the primary source of dependency is encountered.[7] Thus, a change in a personal codependent relationship at home (a husband with alcoholism being hospitalized) may result in an increase in codependent behavior that is noticeable at work.

GUIDELINES FOR THE NURSE MANAGER'S RESPONSE

Some codependent behaviors are mild and require no reaction from the manager. When codependency is situational, that is, related to unusual stress at home or work, the manager may provide temporary support for the stress of the situation.

At other times intervention is necessary. It is important for the manager to be aware that codependent behavior can be adapted and unlearned, and individuals can be helped to form healthy relationships with others. A manager's response to codependency in the workplace, to individuals who act codependently to the manager, or to individuals who are codependent to coworkers or administrators can significantly impact the emotional environment of the workplace. To intervene effectively with problematic codependency the nurse manager should:

- be knowledgeable of codependent behaviors,
- assess the need for intervention when codependent behaviors are present,
- confront nonproductive and detrimental codependent behavior,
- promote positive self concepts,
- facilitate feelings of personal control, and
- refer for counseling or other assistance when indicated.

Be knowledgeable of codependent behaviors

The ongoing acquisition of information that can improve one's personal ability to lead

others is a characteristic of a successful manager.[8] In this case, when the manager has an understanding of codependency, of the typical patterns of codependent behaviors that may be evident in the workplace, and of the factors that motivate codependent behavior, optimal response will be more likely. Information can be acquired by reading or by attending seminars, workshops, or conferences.

Assess need for intervention when codependent behaviors are present

A variety of behaviors may indicate that an employee is codependent. It is easy to respond to the codependent employee with annoyance or anger. Thus the manager's personal anger may be the first indication that a problem exists. In other cases, codependency becomes apparent when coworkers indicate dislike and rejection for the employee who puts in more time than other workers and who keeps reminding others of superior contributions. The overzealous employee may also become noticeable when the manager becomes concerned that the employee will "burn out." Codependency may be present when an employee makes the manager look bad to the manager's supervisor since the employee's performance is more outstanding than the manager's. When major problems in functioning occur and codependent behaviors harm the individual or lead to overwhelming feelings of low self-esteem, intervention may be necessary. When no intervention occurs by the manager, the morale and motivation of the entire work group can be damaged and the manager may end up feeling inadequate and ineffectual.

Confront nonproductive and detrimental codependent behavior

A kind but firm and consistent approach by the manager can assist a codependent individual to decrease self-defeating codependent behavior. "I'm the only one that has this much to do," "I've been here every morning at 6:30," or "I don't think I can stay in a job with these kind of expectations," should not prompt the manager to change or reduce expectations for one employee over another. On the other hand, comments such as "We never get any feedback on what we do," or "I don't know if this is what you want or not," while said in order to elicit direction, indicate to the manager that insecurities are present and more direction is needed.

Promote positive self-concept

Since self-esteem and self-concept are at the core of feelings of codependency, it is important that the manager provide positive feedback to the employee about performance. Positive feedback may be provided orally, in writing, and in front of others when so indicated. Praise and affirmation should be concrete and related to specific actions: "I appreciate the very fine work you did in recruitment this year for nurses; you really had a significant impact on our recruitment problems."

Memos of appreciation may be given directly to the employee or may be copied to the personnel file or the administrator: "I was very impressed with your talk to the Ostomy Club members on home care. You positively represented the professional nursing staff of this hospital to this group and the questions showed that you were helpful to the group members in understanding self care."

The manager may acknowledge the nurse in front of others, for example, in a nursing meeting: "I want to thank Miss Smith for her very fine talk to the Ostomy Club on nursing care issues involved with home care. She was not only willing to come in on her off duty time but put a lot of effort in posters and overheads. If any of you know of another group that would like to hear this talk she has an excellent presentation put together." Trust for the manger will be increased when the manager is consistent and affirming.

Facilitate feelings, personal control

Hospital environments are bureaucratic and encourage codependency by encouraging rigidity, emphasis of rules, and frequent inconsistent enforcement of rules. The typical chain-of-command structure with reward for approved behaviors tends to promote codependence on managers. Helping others, focusing on details, minimizing mistakes, and strict adherence to technical policies and procedures are organizational characteristics of health care agencies that tend to reinforce codependent behaviors.[12] Traditionally managers assumed responsibility for "fixing" problems, thus making employees dependent on managers and leaving managers firmly in control. Unfortunately, some managers have reacted to this system by themselves becoming codependent on the staffs they supervise. This has been especially noted among new managers who lack preparation for their role and vacillate between permissiveness and excessive control and by managers who are required to enforce unpopular policy and blame others for the lack of control: "I can't do anything about it, they are doing it to us again."[12(p.34)]

Since the codependent person has a need to control, when the manager uses a suggestive

---

Trust for the manager will be increased when the manager is consistent and affirming.

---

approach and facilitates feelings of individual control, security can be increased. "I was thinking that if you did it like this, there would be certain advantages . . . what are your thoughts on this?" When a suggestive approach is used, the manager provides direction while at the same time assisting the employee to provide input and to feel in control. "I wonder what you think of doing it like. . . ?" "I know you have the most experience with this and can give me good input. What do you think?" It is important to give the codependent specific achievable tasks that can be done relatively autonomously. While the manager should oversee what is done, direction can be minimal and given only when absolutely necessary. On the other hand, it is important to monitor the codependent since difficulty with ego boundaries may prompt more to be done than the manager wishes.

Allowing staff to participate in management decisions and the initiation of co-governance organizational structures is another way to emphasize the control that staff have over their own destiny. As nurses become empowered and thus are able to exert more control over health care provision, the profession and autonomy of nursing will grow.

Refer for counseling or other assistance when indicated

If the codependent is demonstrating serious performance problems on the job, the employee may need to be referred to an agency or outside counseling service. Even though the manager may be a nurse, this does not mean that diagnosis and treatment should be personally undertaken. The role of the manager is to supervise and not to provide

personal therapy. If an employee assistance program (EAP) is available, the manager should be cognizant of how these services are accessed and should refer the employee. If performance is seriously impaired, it may be necessary to document the referral for the employee's file as a part of a counseling memo: "Employee was counseled about the need to obtain assistance for problems which are affecting performance and was referred to the company EAP." There should be subsequent follow-up to determine if action has been taken by the employee.

•   •   •

Codependence is an important human disorder that is disturbingly prevalent.[1] When codependence is viewed as a psychological concept, it offers a useful framework for evaluating and responding to problematic behavior.

While nursing the addicted and codependent patient and family is an emerging specialty that is helping address the national health care problem of addictions, until now the nursing literature has provided little assistance with the need to recognize codependency from a broad perspective in nursing management. This field offers important and unexplored terrain for the creative and scholarly nurse to assist in developing nursing knowledge. This article has summarized key information about the general problem of codependency and suggests how to apply this information to the setting of the nurse manager. When a nurse manager responds to codependent behavior with understanding and firm control, feelings of security for codependent individuals can be increased and optimum performance will be facilitated.

REFERENCES

1. Cermak, T. *Diagnosing and Treating Co-dependency.* Minneapolis, Minn.: Johnson Institute Books, 1986.
2. American Psychiatric Association. *Diagnostic and Statistical Manual of Mental Disorders,* 3d edition. Washington, D.C.: APA, 1980.
3. Friel, J., Subby, R., and Friel, L. "Co-dependency and the Search for Identity." In *Co-dependence: An Emerging Issue.* Pompano Beach, Fla.: Health Communications, Inc., 1984.
4. Beattie, M. *Co-dependent No More.* Minneapolis, Minn.: Hazelden Foundation, 1987.
5. Whitfield, C. (1987). *Healing the Child Within.* Pompano Beach, Fla.: Health Communications, Inc., 1987.
6. Norwood, R. *Women Who Love Too Much.* Los Angeles, Calif.: Jeremy P. Tarcher, Inc., 1985.
7. Zerwekh, J., and Michaels, B. "Co-dependency." *Nursing Interventions for Addicted Patients* 24, no. 1 (1989): 109–120.
8. Kolenda, M.K. "Co-dependency in the Workplace." *Executive Journal* (July 1989): 37–38.
9. Subby, R. "Inside the Chemically Dependent Marriage: Denial and Manipulation." In *Co-dependence: An Emerging Issue.* Pompano Beach, Fla.: Health Communications, Inc., 1984.
10. Cowan, B., and Gorman, B. "Codependency." *Helplines* (Summer 1990). Ft. Wayne, Ind.: Parkview Memorial Hospital.
11. Wegscheider-Cruse, S. "Co-dependency: The Therapeutic Void." In *Co-dependence: An Emerging Issue.* Pompano Beach, Fla.: Health Communications, Inc., 1984.
12. Cauthorne-Lindstrom, C., and Hrabe, D. "Co-dependent Behaviors in Managers: A Script for Failure." *Nursing Management* 21, no. 2 (1990): 34–9.
13. Mellody, P., Miller, A., and Miller, J. *Facing Codependence: What It Is, Where It Comes From, How It Sabotages Our Lives.* New York, N.Y.: Harper, 1989.

Appendix
Behavioral characteristics of codependents

Five behaviors that may indicate the presence of a potentially damaging codependent were outlined by Kolenda.[8] These behaviors may be noted in the health care setting by the following actions:

1. Enabling. This person tries to cover up the mistakes of others, for example, tardiness or late completion of assignments. A "mother-hen" attitude is communicated: "I'll take care of you because you are incompetent. Besides, I can do it better than you can." While this effort may appear to be good-will on the part of the codependent, it may allow the person who is covered up for to manipulate the manager and the work system. Since actual performance is disguised, it may be difficult for the manager to evaluate individual productivity.

2. Problem hider. Since the codependent person wants to look good and keep things running harmoniously, problems may not be reported until they reach crisis proportions. An attitude of "Let's all be happy! There are no problems here!" is communicated. The manager may have an uneasy feeling that important data are not being reported. While well-intentioned, this behavior can deter intervention until it can no longer be made in a timely manner.

3. Moody. A person who is codependent often appears moody. Since the codependent has a difficult time expressing and analyzing feelings, when asked about the reason for the feelings the answer is often noncommittal and vague. On the other hand this person may be seen as a troublemaker: "I'm going to shake things up around here. They'll be sorry they treated me this way."

4. Poor team player. Since codependents often struggle to please others while at the same time being rigid and inflexible, they often have trouble demonstrating the team spirit necessary for healthy change in a work group. The concern for sameness results in feelings of conflict when change becomes necessary. An attitude of "Leave me alone and I'll do just fine" may be communicated.

5. Burned out. Since codependent individuals have trouble handling feelings they are more prone to stress-related problems. Psychological illnesses related to stress may include, for example, anxiety, insomnia, and hyperactivity. Physical illness related to stress is also likely to be noted, for example, ulcers, hypertension, chemical dependency, migraine headaches, and gastrointestinal disorders.

When the manager encounters "We can't do it!"

Ruth Davidhizar, R.N., D.N.S., C.S.
Assistant Dean and Chair for Nursing
Bethel College
Mishawaka, Indiana

Margaret Bowen, R.N., B.S.N.
Former Assistant Director of Nursing
Logansport State Hospital
Logansport, Indiana

ALL TOO FREQUENTLY nurse managers encounter staff who react to assignments with, "We can't do it!" The manager may be asking to have all nursing care plans updated in a timeframe that staff view as unreasonable. The request may be to change the way dirty linens are sent to the laundry when staff feel the resources needed to correct this problem are beyond their control. The manager's direction may be for attendance at an inservice training session in addition to completing multiple patient care assignments.

"We can't do it!" is sometimes said to the manager at the time the direction is given. In other cases, the negative response is indirect and becomes apparent by a delay in starting the assignment, by intentional inefficiency in doing the assignment, or by failure to complete the assigned task. Regardless of whether the resistive response is direct or indirect, "We can't do it!" represents a variety of dynamics. An "I can't do it!" response may be motivated

Health Care Superv, 1992, 11(1), 27–32
©1992 Aspen Publishers, Inc.

by hostility, the desire to get back at authority, a generally negative personality, or feelings of helplessness or powerlessness. When a negative response is precipitated by a feeling of powerlessness, the nurse manager faces a challenging interpersonal dilemma. On the other hand, a "We can't do it" response may indicate a cohesive group phenomenon or an effort to utilize the group for support. Resistance in a group presents additional challenges to the manager. This article addresses this dilemma by describing the relationship of powerlessness to a negative response and the unique problems of negative responses in a group setting. Presented will be intervention strategies that may be used by the nurse manager to decrease feelings of powerlessness and strategies to use when responding to nurses who act negatively in a group setting.

POWERLESSNESS

Personal

Power can be defined in many ways. Webster indicates it is "the possession of control, authority, or influence over others."[1] Power is an evocative word that frequently conjures up negative feelings. This is unfortunate since power pervades all aspects of organizational life and nurses need an understanding of power and how to use it if they are to succeed in their organizational goals. Even more important to nursing success than an understanding of power, however, is an understanding of the incapacitating feeling of powerlessness.

Perhaps more than any other professionals, nurses must deal with situations that cannot be controlled.[2] Powerlessness is an intrinsic part of the health care setting in which professionals respond to life-threatening situations. Nurses helping patients face death for the first time often worry that there was something else they could have done. Sleepless nights and anxiety may be experienced. However, most nurses overcome the initial feeling of being overwhelmed and accept the human limitations that often exist in a life-threatening situation. Some degree of powerlessness is accepted as part of being a nurse.

In addition to the powerlessness experienced when human actions cannot avert the course of death, powerlessness is often experienced by nurses in response to their perceived inability to change problems in the health care system. In the present day health care setting, nurses are being asked to do more with less, that is, less staff, less resources, and less time. In this crisis-oriented health care climate, feelings of powerlessness and "We can't do it!" responses may be expected.

Health care system problems that create feelings of persisting powerlessness are frequently interpersonal. While powerlessness over death is more likely to be accepted, powerlessness over people may cause ongoing personal turmoil. Powerlessness over people or the perceived inability to affect problems related to the health care system is often further compounded by feelings of personal inadequacy. Yet another issue is that feelings of powerlessness in the health care system, rather than being primarily system-imposed, are also significantly affected by personal perceptions. For example, while two nurses may be involved in the same situation, one may react by being overwhelmed while the other may proceed undaunted.

In circumstances that cannot be controlled, powerlessness may be inevitable. Consider, for example, a staff member who becomes ill and has no means to support the family.

However, for the most part, feelings of powerlessness are the result of feelings of inadequacy resulting from interpersonal disharmony, a situation that induces stress, and the perception an individual has of a situation.

In a group

When persons state feelings of powerlessness in a group, additional issues must be considered. The individual may reflect the feelings of the majority of the group. On the other hand, the individual may be the only one who has that particular feeling and may not speak for the group at large. The stated feelings may or may not describe the intensity of the feelings of the members of the group.

Negative feelings may be spoken in a group in order to elicit support and when none is given, the feelings may be laid aside. On the other hand, if support is felt, momentum can be gained to increase the strength of the resistance. A "We can't do it" statement in a group may cause some members who had not considered this position to take sides and also become resistive.

A "We can't do it" statement is often meant to manipulate the manager to change or decrease expectations. One benefit of a negative response in a group setting is that the manager may be less inclined to publicly disagree and may therefore go along with the stated position. In the hope of eliciting a different response in a group, some employ-

---

A "We can't do it" statement in a group may cause some members who had not considered this position to take sides and also become resistive.

---

ees may ask a question to which the manager has already responded in a previous one-to-one encounter. Additionally, the individual who needs group support feels braver in a group and more willing to state a feeling that the others may share.

INTERVENTION STRATEGIES

A manager should carefully plan intervention strategies intended to deter negative responses. In addition, a manager needs strategies that assist individuals in dealing with feelings of powerlessness. Finally, managers need to have skill in handling individuals and groups when powerless feelings are stated in a group setting. Intervention strategies should include communicating a positive expectation, increasing feelings of self-worth, timing assignments strategically, involving staff actively in problem solving, and providing staff with information. Finally, setting limits to negative responses in a group is crucial in skillful management of staff.

Positive expectations

In some situations, feelings of powerlessness are related to the approach of the manager. If the manager assertively indicates the expectation that change *will* occur, the manager's positive expectation may avert a reaction of powerlessness and a "We can't do it!" response. A manager with a known reputation for setting limits on manipulative behavior and for not tolerating resistance will often receive less resistance.[3] On the other hand, a manager whose tone is tentative or uncertain will be more likely to receive negative reactions from staff. If the manager is known to be easily influenced by the staff's negative reactions, staff are much more likely to resist instruction that is disliked.

Skillful questioning is one positive way to persuade people to accept change and to respond to direction.[3] Communication that frames questions to invite affirmative responses, for example, "Wouldn't you agree that . . ." or "Wouldn't it be helpful to . . ." capitalize upon establishing hopeful, affirmative attitudes toward desired changes. With positive questioning the manager's opinion is clearly articulated and there is no uncertainty that the manager wants the staff member to share the perspective. A positive question that invites a one word affirmative answer is more likely to elicit a "Yes" response.[3]

Increase feelings of self-worth

The manager who has established rapport with personnel and who recognizes ability is more likely to receive a positive response when assignments are given. Everyone wants to feel recognized, important, and valued.[4] These needs are powerful motivators for increased performance and positive feelings about assignments. When nursing staff are recognized and rewarded for what they do, they are much more likely to be cooperative.

In a study by Reece and Brandt, positive written communication, while noted to be generally underutilized, was found to be a very important motivating factor for employees.[5] Pinder also identified that how employees are perceived by others has a significant effect on job satisfaction, productivity, and self-perception.[6] Others have noted employee productivity will be increased in order to maintain that positive feeling.[7] In a study by Graham and Unruh, it was noted that the techniques that had the greatest impact are "manager initiated" and "performance based" and include such methods as verbal praise, personal notes, public recogni-

tion, special privileges, and pictures and notes on bulletin boards.[4(p.9)] It was also noted that such techniques, while they are least costly, tend to be used less frequently than other more expensive motivational techniques, for example, employee-of-the-month plaques, turkeys on holidays, and hats and mugs with agency logo.

Promote feelings of personal power

Nurses derive power not from their agencies or their positions but from their personalities.[2(p.103)] In fact, it has been said that success in nursing is related less to knowledge than to a strong sense of personal power.[8] Since feelings of power are primarily personal rather than "organizational," feelings of power can be influenced by the manager. A manager can indicate to staff that they have power by using words, actions, and attitudes that give staff feelings of control. For example "Do you want to do it like— or—?," giving staff the feeling that they are choosing their actions may make disagreeable tasks more palatable. A manager can also assist staff to see the positive aspects of negative situations; for example, "You'll know what to do next time" or "Aren't we lucky that we will have to do this only once?"

While it is important for personal feelings of power to be experienced in relation to the job setting, nurses need a strong sense of self-worth based on who they are in their own right.[9] When nurses fulfill organizational demands at the expense of not taking care of themselves, the institutional authority determines the worth of the nurse as a person. Internalization of the institutional authority's appraisal of individual worth can lead to feelings of inadequacy. Nurses need to be responsible to themselves first and to their employer second. A nurse who can use a sense of humor rather than taking the job too seriously may be able to see the humor in the incongruencies of the job setting.

Utilize strategic timing

Another managerial attribute that may trigger a negative response is unreasonable or poorly timed demands. If a manager's assignments exceed what staff feel can reasonable be done in the time available, or are timed when staff already feel overworked or frustrated, a negative reaction is more likely to occur. Feelings of powerlessness are also intensified and often mushroom when several individuals who feel powerless are together as a work group or when an assignment is given. In other words, the strategy of the manager in how and to whom assignments are given is another factor in reducing or increasing feelings of powerlessness in a group. The manager who arranges the environment in a positive way is more likely to promote and foster success. If a negative reaction is expected to an assignment, it is better to elicit support by approaching individually those persons expected to be negative. An individual approach is more likely to be convincing since a personal approach communicates respect and concern.

Involve staff in problem solving

Powerlessness in the face of problems in the agency system is aggravated when staff feel they have been excluded from input into problem solving and planning concerning what are perceived as significant job-related issues. Powerless feelings are also stimulated when staff feel they are not recognized or respected for what they do. Staff who perceive they have not been rewarded for their efforts are more likely to respond negatively when assignments are given.

Research from the business world indicates that participative management influences and promotes positive outcome.[10] The nursing literature as well has suggested the need to involve nurses in decision making.[8(p.334)] Adequate control over the practice of nursing (professional autonomy) and the structuring of work (job autonomy) contribute to the feeling of pride in what is done.

Prescott and Dennis suggest that the power of individual nurses and the power of the nursing department is a largely underdeveloped resource.[8] Involving nurses in policy making meetings can both strengthen the satisfaction of nurses and can increase the effective delivery of nursing service. It is important for nurse managers to be aware that internal derisiveness weakens the collective power of the nursing department.[8] Upgrading the educational preparation and administrative sophistication of head nurses also adds to increasing the power savvy of nurses at the unit level. When nurses are active in policy formation and decision making in the organization, their self-respect is increased.

Increase staff knowledge of health care system

Information can be a powerful defense against feelings of powerlessness. Providing staff with information about their job in orientation and in ongoing training can equip staff to respond assertively rather than to be confused and hesitant. Adequate direction is related to attaining organizational goals.

Feeling of powerlessness are often precipitate not by planned actions of another, but by accidents of the organization.[2] For example, an assignment to inservice training by the inservice director who has little awareness of the actual staffing of the nursing care unit may trigger powerlessness. When staff understand the source of apparently random and illogical actions and know what recourse is available to them, action can be taken and feelings of powerlessness can be decreased or eliminated. Understanding the dynamics and the facts that have gone into decisions about assignments may make an unpalatable decision more palatable.

Set limits on negativism

When a statement is made in a group setting indicating powerlessness, such as "I can't do it" or "We can't do it," it is beneficial to say, "I'll discuss that with you later, we need to use the group time to decide on . . ." One individual's feelings of powerlessness can be transmitted to others in a group setting if limit setting does not occur. A manager who is unable to control the focus of discussion in a group may add to the feeling of powerlessness in the group because of the perception that the manager is not in control.

Humor may also be used to limit negative feelings in a group. For example, "You are asking for logic when logic died and was buried last week" can both give the indi-

vidual recognition and minimize the negative effect of the comments.

• • •

This article has described the importance of increasing staff feelings of self-worth, of promoting feelings of personal power, involving staff actively in practice issues, of increasing staff knowledge of the health care and agency system, and of setting limits on negative discussion in a group. When nurses feel power in the health care system, it not only has the benefit of increasing job satisfaction but increases positive responses on the job.[11] On the other hand, nursing staff who are unable to conquer the feeling of powerlessness may respond to assignments with statements signifying the subjective state experienced: "We can't do it!" Such staff are unlikely to experience personal and professional rewards and may ultimately leave the health care field. This negative process may be blocked by the manager who assists staff to develop feelings of worth, professional autonomy, and control and who can appropriately handle negative feelings expressed in a group.

REFERENCES

1. *Webster's New Collegiate Dictionary.* Springfield, Mass.: G & C Merriam Co., 1984.
2. Korobow, L., Smith, R., and Kushel, G. "Think You're Powerless? Think again." *Nursing* 89 (1989): 103–9.
3. Davidhizar, R., and Bowen, M. "Confrontation: An Underused Nursing Management Technique." *Health Care Supervisor* 7, no. 1 (1988): 29–34.
4. Graham, G., and Unruh, J. "The Motivational Impact of Nonfinancial Employee Appreciation Practices on Medical Technologists." *Health Care Supervisor* 8, no. 3 (1990): 9–17.
5. Reece, B.L., and Brandt, R. *Effective Human Relations in Organizations,* 2nd ed. Englewood Cliffs, N.J.: Prentice Hall, 1982.
6. Pinder, C. *Work Motivation: Theory, Issues and Applications.* New York, N.Y.: Scott Foresman, 1984.
7. Reber, R.W., and Van Gilder, G. *Behavioral Insights for Supervision,* 2nd ed. Englewood Cliffs, N.J.: Prentice Hall, 1982.
8. Prescott, P., and Dennis, K. "Power and Powerlessness in Hospital Nursing Departments." *Journal of Professional Nursing* 1, no. 6: 334-55.
9. Tomey, A. "President's Report." *ISNA Bulletin* 16, no. 6 (1990): 1.
10. Goddard, R.W. "Motivating the Modern Employee." *Management World* 13, no. 2 (1984): 8–10.
11. Inlander, C. "The Fight against Powerlessness." *Nursing and Health Care* 9, no. 9 (1988): 385–6.

Managing organizational aversion among health care workers

Howard L. Smith
Consulting Research Scientist

Neill F. Piland
Director
Health Services Research and Education
Lovelace Medical Foundation
Albuquerque, New Mexico

DURING THE LAST decade, revisions in reimbursement policy; aggressive competition; multiinstitutional system development; expanding corporate influence, diversification, and joint ventures; and a more enlightened consumer constituency have seriously challenged health care professionals.[1] The catalyst producing these pressures has been the development of multiinstitutional systems.[2] While large-scale organizations provide distinct advantages for achieving economies of scale, they also present disadvantages that may affect personnel. Concern about the dysfunctions accompanying large-scale health care organizations is most noticeable among clinicians (e.g., physicians and nurses).[3,4] However, health care supervisors may also have observed uneasiness among staff members about the power and control of health care organizations. The implications of this trend are critical to health care supervisors: if personnel become distracted,

Health Care Superv, 1989, 7(4), 1–10
© 1989 Aspen Publishers, Inc.

they are less able to provide effective services or to maintain productivity.

Harmony between personnel and an organization can be disrupted by any number of factors. Compensation, performance expectations, lack of employee participation in decision making, and deficient leadership are a few examples. Many of the characteristics of large-scale organizations create disharmony—organizational aversion among employees. In its most basic form, organizational aversion makes personnel reluctant to sincerely commit to an organization or its goals.[5,6] Workers may hesitate to cooperate with employers because they sense an inherent struggle between them and their organization. Organizational aversion among health care workers threatens productivity, efficiency, and quality of care. If personnel do not sanction organizational efforts, they may render their work units and departments less effective in achieving goals, which, in turn, undermines health care organizations' efforts to address environmental constraints such as prospective payment, competition, or corporate takeover threats.[7]

Organizational aversion has many similarities to patterns of alienation.

To promote the desire of health care personnel to work within a supportive organization, supervisors must provide the proper milieu, circumventing the pressures that create conflicts between personnel and organizations.[8-10] In short, supervisors must manage the contention that generates a feeling of organizational aversion among their staff members. By reducing the contention between staff and organization, supervisors can create opportunities for employee and organizational growth.

The purposes of this article are to define the concept of organizational aversion, explain how it is becoming more prevalent in health care organizations, and examine specific methods of minimizing organizational aversion.

ORGANIZATIONAL AVERSION AND ITS CAUSES

Organizational aversion is an adverse reaction by personnel to growing organizational control over their lives and work that threatens the interrelationship of personnel and organizations. Health care personnel are aware of their limited impact on strategic decisions and plans.[11] They are excluded from strategic-level decisions that determine how organizations operate, under what policies, with guidance from which strategic objectives, and with what degree of resource support. Health care employees may feel unable to contribute in significant ways to organizations. They may perceive that their roles are considered to be inconsequential to the larger service delivery process.

Organizational aversion has many similarities to patterns of alienation. Supervisors should be alert for symptoms of organizational aversion:

- consistent cynicism or pessimism about organizational values, operations, and issues;
- disagreement with the goals established for work units, departments, and the organization;
- hesitancy to cooperate with other personnel or departments outside of immediate work unit;

- resistance to proposed changes; and
- emphasis on self-interest rather than team effort.

Supervisors should suspect organizational aversion whenever they detect a general climate of disagreement and resistance to organizationally based efforts.

Circumstances causing organizational aversion include

- exclusion of operating-level personnel's participation in or contribution to strategy formulation and objective-setting processes;
- limited channels of communication from operating level to top management;
- upward flow of information without reciprocity from top management;
- introduction of major organizational changes (e.g., staff reductions) without preparing staff;
- concentration of power and control in top management or corporate offices;
- use of organizational methods to promote growth in service delivery; and
- revision of goals to emphasize efficiency, profitability, and market share at the expense of patients and personnel.

When these causes exist, personnel are somewhat powerless to alter the basic relationship between them and their employer. Staff may feel unable to correct significant obvious problems in service delivery. Few communication channels to top management are available to employees. In short, employees feel devalued and that their concerns exist in a vacuum. Meanwhile, the importance of the organization grows inversely to the importance of staff.

Supervisors, caught in the middle of this conflict, can either ignore the problem or address the symptoms and causal factors. Inaction will mean an escalating problem that may erupt with severe consequences (high absenteeism, high turnover, and union activity), or, under more fortunate circumstances, top management will recognize the problem and administer organizationwide solutions. Alternatively, supervisors can manage the problem by creating a better climate for staff members and patients or clients. To formulate an effective treatment program, supervisors must understand what causes organizational aversion.

Organizational intensity in health care

Although organizational aversion has always been present in the health care field, its intensity has been minimal because of the prevailing cost-based reimbursement systems, the nonprofit orientation of health care providers, and the lack of multiinstitutional arrangements among health care organizations. Health care has traditionally been delivered through low-stress, resource-rich, nonsystematized institutions whose mission was primarily patient service. This tradition has been replaced by an entrepreneurial, competitive, and multiinstitutional industry that pursues diverse goals. This change has resulted in four situations that alter the role of health care workers, even physicians.

Central to the changing health care field are new organization cultures that emphasize efficiency, economies of scale, and return on investment.[12] This new emphasis may produce an organization culture that employees find less than gratifying.

First, profit has become a legitimate organizational goal. Inevitably, quality of care clashes with profit (or efficiency). However, neither organizations nor health care professionals have been able to determine the extent to which quality should be traded for profit or efficiency and vice versa. As a result, health care organizations blindly try to achieve both quality and profit without understanding the consequences of mutually conflicting goals. Inevitably, staff suffer the brunt of this conflict.

Second, multiinstitutional systems have expanded in health care.[13] Systems of care, as well as systems comprised of smaller systems, have proliferated in the health care environment. Multiinstitutional alliances, arrangements, and systems are developing among formerly autonomous providers. The end result is that employees find themselves at the bottom of a very complex organizational structure, their institutions representing only one unit within a larger system of institutions.[14] Power is no longer locally based but is centralized in corporate offices, possibly in another state, and invested in individuals whose names, faces, ideals, or agendas are not well known.

Third, control of health care organizations is concentrated in the hands of professional managers whose frame of reference is organizational well-being.[15] These managers, responsible for chains or systems of organizations, may be sympathetic to the plight of any single institution, but their allegiance is to the system as a whole. This orientation may conflict with clinical and nonclinical staff orientation. The inherent altruism of health care delivery is being replaced by a new set of goals in which employees have little voice. Consistent with this change, employees are viewed as productive resources. Management attempts to derive the maximum productivity for a given investment from these resources.

Fourth, as diversification has increased

among health care providers, many organizations have lost their identities.[16,17] The scope of corporate strategy has broadened until virtually any link to health services makes a business opportunity a legitimate strategic option. Many health care organizations are experimenting with services in which they lack a competitive advantage. Furthermore, diversification has obscured the traditional purpose of health care. Staff observe that the values of new personnel groups are not necessarily the same values as those of dominant culture. Personnel also recognize that any service area, including their own, is now potentially expendable.

Organizational aversion has become more prominent with the growth of health care organizational forces. The prognosis is that organizational influence will intensify as health care providers wrestle with the complex pressures present in the health care sector. The implications for employees are numerous, and many conflicts between personnel and organizations are likely in the foreseeable future. Health care supervisors will be confronted by these conflicts unless their institutions establish specific plans and actions for neutralizing the forces of contention.

The organizational imperative

The trend toward increased organizational influence in society has been termed the organizational imperative.[18] According to this view, organizations dominate many aspects of life, particularly the production of goods and services.[19] Experts argue that several fundamental value shifts accompany this growth of the organizational imperative. Ideals of individuality; spontaneity; a sense of community, indispensability, and self-worth are being lost to ideals of obedience, control, planning, paternalism, dispensability, and organizational worth. Employees hold the former value set while organizations pursue the latter. When organizational values dominate at the expense of employee values, personnel feel organizational aversion. Managers and supervisors can help employees overcome this aversion and temper the excesses of organization at the operating level by treating individuals with dignity and emphasizing their worth as individuals.

Given the trends toward organizational intensity in the health care field, the presence of the organizational imperative is not unanticipated. An underlying belief at health care strategic management levels is that the best interests of health care can be achieved primarily through organizations.[20] This attitude ultimately affects staff members: growth in organizational preeminence corresponds to devaluation of individual workers. This is particularly true for occupations in which labor supply is high or demand for labor is low. Because many of the ancillary service positions in health care organizations meet these criteria, supervisors can anticipate organizational aversion among staff members.

Conflicts between individual and organizational goals

Organizational aversion reaches significant proportions when the goals of individuals and the goals of organizations diverge.[21,22] Employees are motivated to join organizations for reasons other than just to be employed and to earn compensation. They may be attracted to a particular health care organization because it has a reputation for high-quality care, exceptional customer or patient service, a renowned medical staff, opportunities for employee growth, profit sharing, or other salient attractions.[23] Staff are disappointed to discover that organizations are ignoring those motives.[24] When their values are not recognized, employees are left with few other choices than to terminate their affiliation or to respond in counterproductive ways.[25,26]

Even nonprofit organizations are beginning to mimic their for-profit counterparts, emphasizing financial statement bottom lines and becoming more reluctant to support amenities or financially constrained operations than in the past. Nonprofits must emulate for-profit organizations if they intend to survive financially. Consequently, most health care organizations are cultivating a climate in which organizational aversion is possible.

The reorientation of organizational goals is alarming to staff members who have not adopted, or do not have the incentives to adopt, a new philosophy for health care delivery. Furthermore, employees who have traditionally held very little power or prestige in organizations are witnessing an even greater deterioration of their status. In the end, many health care workers are left frustrated with their occupations and their organizations. Once part of a noble effort, health care workers are discovering that they are very similar to employees in manufacturing sectors. Service delivery is scrutinized for the consumption of resources and production of revenue. Employees are essential, yet expendable, units of production.

The lack of harmony between individual goals and organizational goals is more than just a disquieting disconformity. While health care organizations are adopting new goals, they are also asking health care workers to work even harder. For example, nurses directly confront the demands of resource-constrained organizations.[27] Decreasing expensive nurse staffing is often the easiest way to trim costs in the short run but places a greater burden on remaining nurses to provide high-quality, nurturing care to patients. Simultaneously, health care institutions are requesting further assistance in meeting cost control goals. Squeezed to the limit, nurses and other health care workers not surprisingly have difficulty in joining the drive toward greater austerity. Such tactics may not be consistent with their view of how services or care should be delivered. Moreover, they recognize that the next level of staffing cuts may slash their positions. Under these circumstances, one can understand why employees are not embracing organizational goals.

Management theory and research suggest that the best organizations provide a culture in which the organization and its personnel share the same values, beliefs, attitudes, and goals.[28,29] When these cultures are working, remarkable gains can be made in productivity, quality, costs, and profit.[30] Because organizational aversion is counterproductive to an effective culture, organizations and managers must address the goal conflict that causes organizational aversion.

METHODS FOR MINIMIZING ORGANIZATIONAL AVERSION

As Figure 1 suggests, increasing organizational intensity in health care, combined with prevailing trends in organizational climates, creates the need to minimize organizational aversion. The most

frequently mentioned remedy in health care literature is to encourage accommodation between organization and employees.[31-33] Both organization and staff members must appreciate the other's goals and values in order to create an effective service delivery environment.

Management theory and research suggest that the best organizations provide a culture in which the organization and its personnel share the same values, beliefs, attitudes, and goals.

How can the concept of accommodation be effectively implemented? Available research suggests three promising strategies for reaching a mutual understanding and collaborative relationship between organizations and employees: anticipation, diagnosis, and treatment.[34] Organizations and supervisors, invested with the power to revise the infrastructure and service delivery process, are responsible for initiating these strategies. In contrast, employees have relatively little power to initiate change, especially when their goals differ fundamentally from organization goals. As a result, organizations must take the lead in resolving differences.

Anticipation

Organizations must be more sensitive to the impact of their decisions, plans, and changes on employees. Staff members who ultimately implement changes in an organization often find the prospect of undertaking change traumatic. Therefore, supervisors

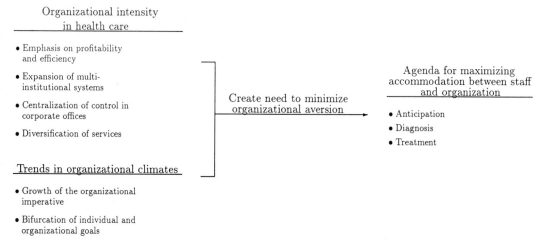

Figure 1. Formulating strategies to minimize organizational aversion.

must anticipate and minimize the dysfunctional consequences resulting from operational changes. Anticipation may mean simply soliciting input from staff members when a change is being considered. Staff might be asked to recommend methods for minimizing adverse effects on patients and personnel. If supervisors seek staff input before planning and implementing changes, staff members are more likely to be committed to successfully implementing plans. When input is not solicited, decisions or actions may be viewed as unilateral and organizationally centered.

In other situations, anticipation may mean keeping staff members informed of pending decisions or plans and the rationale for such actions. The key is to expand communications to prevent the possibility of miscommunication or misinterpretation. For example, supervisors can brief staff on the progress of new projects so that employees understand why certain events are happening and what direction will be taken in the future. The communication

should not be one sided. Staff should be encouraged to analyze the impact of specific changes on departmental or work unit operations. Recommendations for improving changes conceived by other managers can also be solicited. Through this sharing, miscommunication can be avoided and commitment elicited.

Diagnosis

Organizational aversion is easily detected when health care supervisors remain alert to its potential outbreak. However, supervisors are often hesitant to probe too far when they discover dissatisfaction among staff members. They may perceive that personnel do not want any intrusion, or they may not know how to resolve problems and so hesitate to pursue the matter further. Supervisors with these attitudes risk compounding problems. Detecting and treating problems is difficult unless the extent of the issue is clarified. By prudent assessment and incorporating findings into a plan of action, health care supervisors can minimize the growth of organizational aversion.

For example, supervisors might ascertain the extent to which staff members share the same values as the organization. Through personal discussions and group meetings a profile of the value of employees within a work unit or department can be established. In other cases, supervisors may use surveys to assess attitudes. Using this information, supervisors can better understand any difference between organization value and individual, group, work unit, or department values and can make plans for managing the variance. Diagnosis identifies the problem and helps clarify what interventions are needed and for whom, in order to create a healthier environment for staff.

Treatment

Unless supervisors initiate corrective action, organizational aversion may continue to hamper employee performance. Supervisors must recognize that no panacea or quick fix has much promise of resolving the fundamental problem. Instead, a reasonable treatment plan considers the causes of organizational aversion and responds accordingly.

In many cases this means that supervisors will be challenged to help staff members see that equity can be attained between personal aspirations and organizational goals. Commitment can be elicited by creating opportunities for investment on the part of staff members. When they have meaningful input into work unit or department changes, staff are more likely to perceive that the resulting program reflects their goals.

Not every employee wants to participate in determining how organizational changes will take place. Some employees may wish to avoid the issue altogether, and supervisors should anticipate this response. The process of participation acquires a sense of purpose among those employees who do participate. When employees are judiciously approached for their thoughts on work unit or departmental issues, they more readily offer their suggestions, even though they are normally hesitant to do so. In this manner, organizational aversion loses its power because staff have an active role directing their work unit or department. Trust and understanding begin to bridge the gap between individual and organization values.

Another approach is to restructure the delivery process around teams. The purpose of team building is to erase the rigid formality characterizing bureaucratic organizations, creating an environment in which efficiency is desirable but does not exclude broader goals such as effectiveness. Redesigning work units to form collaborative teams or quality circles can forge a spirit of cooperation. As part of a collaborative team rather than a formal work unit, staff are better able to inject their values into the work process.

IMPLICATIONS FOR HEALTH CARE SUPERVISORS

From many perspectives health care organizations seem to be serving their own interests instead of employee interests. In spite of this conflict, organizations and employees obviously depend on each other. Organizations cannot deliver high-quality, low-cost services without committed employees. Conversely, personnel need a work environment that supports their basic value system and dignity; otherwise, they become averse to their job setting. Organizational aversion is a significant issue for health care supervisors, who are in a position to implement remedial strategies that reduce the underlying tension. Through anticipation, diagnosis, and treatment, supervisors can improve the opportunities staff members have to contribute to the evolving goals of organizations.

REFERENCES

1. Kimberly, J.R., and Zajac, E.J. "Strategic Adaptation in Health Care Organizations: Implications for Theory and Research." *Medical Care* 42 (1985): 267–302.

2. Relman, A.S. "The New Medicine-industrial Complex." *New England Journal of Medicine* 303 (1980): 963–70.

3. Shortell, S.M. "The Medical Staff of the Future: Replanting the Garden." *Frontiers of Health Services Management* 1, no. 3 (1985): 3–48.

4. Kralewski, J.E., et al. "The Physician Rebellion." *New England Journal of Medicine* 316 (1985): 339–42.

5. Mowday, R.T., Porter, L.W., and Steers, R.M. *Employee-Organization Linkages: The Psychology of Commitment, Absenteeism and Turnover.* New York. Academic Press, 1982.

6. Argyris, C. *Integrating the Individual and the Organization.* New York: Wiley, 1964.

7. Ermann, D., and Gabel, J. "Multihospital Systems: Issues and Empirical Findings." *Health Affairs* 3, no. 1 (1984): 50-64.

8. Culbert, S.A., and McDonough, J.J. *The Invisible War: Pursuing Self Interests at Work.* New York: Wiley, 1980.

9. Barnard, C.I. *The Function of the Executive.* Cambridge: Harvard University Press, 1938.

10. Katz, D., and Kahn, R.L. *The Social Psychology of Organizations.* New York: Wiley, 1966.

11. Hillman, A.L., et al. "Managing the Medical-industrial Complex." *New England Journal of Medicine* 315 (1986): 511-13.

12. Gray, B.H. "Overview: Origins and Trends." *Bulletin of the New York Academy of Medicine* 61, no. 1 (1985): 7–22.

13. Fottler, M.D., et al. "Multiinstitutional Arrangements in Health Care: Review, Analysis, and a Proposal for Future Research." *Academy of Management Review* 7, no. 1 (1982): 67–69.

14. Brown, M. "Changes in Corporate Organization of the Health Care System." *Health Matrix* 2, no. 1 (1984): 27–30.

15. Quintana, J.B., Duncan, W.J., and Houser, H.W. "Hospital Governance and the Corporate Revolution." *Health Care Management Review* 10, no. 3 (1985): 63–71.

16. Goldsmith, J.C. "Competition: How Will It Affect Hospitals?" *Healthcare Financial Management* 36, no. 1 (1982): 64–74.

17. Finkler, S.A., and Horowitz, S.L. "Merger and Consolidation: An Overview of Activity in Health Care Organizations." *Healthcare Financial Management* 39, no. 1 (1985): 19–26.

18. Scott, W.G., and Hart, K.D. *Organizational America.* Boston: Houghton Mifflin, 1979.

19. Whyte, W.H. *The Organization Man.* New York: Simon & Schuster, 1956.

20. Fottler, M.D. "Health Care Organizational Performance: Present and Future Research." *Journal of Management* 13 (1987): 367–91.

21. Campbell, J.P., et al. *Managerial Behavior, Performance and Effectiveness.* New York: McGraw-Hill, 1970.

22. James, L.R., and Jones, A.P. "Organizational Climate: A Review of Theory and Research." *Psychological Bulletin* 81 (1974): 1096–112.

23. Mowday, R.T., Porter, L.W., and Steers, R.M. *Employee-Organization Linkages: The Psychology of Commitment, Absenteeism and Turnover.* New York: Academic Press, 1982.

24. Smith, C.A., Organ, D.W., and Near, J.P. "Organizational Citizenship Behavior: Its Nature and Antecedents." *Journal of Applied Psychology* 68 (1983): 653–63.

25. Randall, D.M. "Commitment and the Organization: The Organization Man Revisited." *Academy of Management Review* 12 (1987): 460–71.

26. Reichers, A.E. "A Review and Reconceptualization of Organization Commitment." *Academy of Management Review* 10 (1985): 465–76.

27. Inglehart, J.K. "Problems Facing the Nursing Profession." *New England Journal of Medicine* 317 (1987): 646–51.

28. Peters, T.J., and Waterman, R.H. *In Search of Excel-*

lence. New York: Warner Books, 1982.

29. Sathe, V. *Culture and Related Corporate Realities.* Homewood, Ill.: Irwin, 1985.

30. Smircich, L. "Concepts of Culture and Organizational Analysis." *Administrative Science Quarterly* 28 (1983): 339–58.

31. Simendinger, E.A., and Pasmore, W. "Developing Partnerships between Physicians and Health Care Executives." *Hospital and Health Services Admini-* *stration Quarterly* 29, no. 6 (1984): 21–35.

32. Fried, B.J. "Collaboration, Not Co-optation." *Canadian Medical Journal* 135 (1986): 733–36.

33. Scott, W.R. "Managing Professional Work: Three Models of Control for Health Organizations." *Health Services Research* 17 (1982): 213–40.

34. Wright, S., and Wright, A. "A Cooperative Organizational Form for Hospitals." *Health Care Management Review* 9, no. 2 (1984): 7–19.

Part III
Some Special Problems
and Processes

The manager as conflict negotiator

Rita E. Numerof
Assistant Professor
George Warren Brown School of
Social Work
Washington University
St. Louis, Missouri

TYPICALLY, supervisory personnel in health care institutions
are promoted internally. Until fairly
recently, little attention was paid to
training these new managers in the
techniques of management. One un-
written assumption was that the new
supervisor's competence in the technical or clinical area would translate
automatically into managerial competence. Another common assumption
was that where management training
was offered, the focus was often on
the "harder" aspects—staffing, budgeting and planning. The human relations components critical to the processes of motivation, performance
appraisal, coaching and discipline,
were too frequently taken for
granted.

The result of such inattention was
that the negotiation of conflict, probably the most difficult aspect of the
communications process, was also
overlooked. The ramification of such

Health Care Superv, 1985,3(3),1–15
© 1985 Aspen Publishers, Inc.

Interpersonal Roles	Informational Roles	Decisional Roles
• Figurehead • Leader • Liaison	• Monitor • Disseminator • Spokesperson	• Entrepreneur • Disturbance handler • Resource allocator • Negotiator

an oversight in economically sound times is higher turnover. Under conditions of economic restraint, the ramifications are less dramatic but may be seen in poor morale, scapegoating and tensions within the work group, as well as in diminished performance and productivity.

CONFLICT IN MANAGERIAL ROLES

Conflict is an inevitable part of any manager's job. An examination of the key roles of the manager as outlined by Mintzberg highlights this fact.[1] According to Mintzberg, there are ten roles (boxed material), classified as interpersonal, informational or decisional, that a manager plays regardless of position in the organizational hierarchy. How dominant a particular role is will be determined by the nature of the organization—its mission, culture and structure—as well as by the manager's position within that structure.

Interpersonal roles

The interpersonal roles include figurehead, leader and liaison. As a figurehead, the manager performs ceremonial tasks, such as greeting new staff members to the work unit and arranging for their integration. In the capacity of leader, the manager performs some crucial activities that determine supervisory effectiveness. Some of these are direct activities, such as hiring and training. Some are more subtle, such as motivating and providing internal coordination. These activities determine how effectively subordinates will work to accomplish the goals of the group. Not infrequently, discrepancies occur between expectations and accomplishments. Resolving such discrepancies, particularly where subordinates' perceptions of the situation differ from that of the supervisor, necessitates the effective management of conflict.

Conflict is an inevitable part of any manager's job. How dominant a particular manager's role is will be determined by the nature of the organization as well as the manager's position within that structure.

As liaison, the supervisor makes contacts outside the vertical chain of command. Studies of managerial activities have shown that managers spend as much time with peers and others outside their work units as they do with their own subordinates. Middle managers, for example, have been found to spend as much as 47 percent of their time with peers.[2] Although much of the liaison function entails gathering pertinent information from outside the work group, conflict may occur in gaining access to the information. In addition, because no role exists as a distinct entity, conflict may occur as information gathering evolves into issues over turf, and as the manager is perceived (and rightly so) as a spokesperson for a particular work group with vested interests.

Informational roles

Any manager is the hub of interaction within the work group and between that unit and other units. The manager knows more about the unit than any other member of the staff. As monitor, disseminator and spokesperson, much of the manager's job consists of processing this information.

As a monitor, the manager scans the environment for information through a network of peer contacts and subordinates, keeping in touch with the flow of events in the organization. In the role of disseminator, the manager passes some of the privileged information directly to subordinates, who would otherwise not have

access to it. As spokesperson, the manager sends information about the work unit to others outside the unit, for example, via hospitalwide management meetings or by simply keeping superiors informed. Conflict in informational roles may emanate from a variety of sources, for example, through perceived and real lack of access to critical information, or through dissatisfaction with the content or implications of the communication that is shared.

Decisional roles

Information processing is crucial to the last set of roles—the decisional roles. Obviously, the manager plays a major role in the unit's decision-making system. The manager possesses both the formal authority and current information necessary to make effective decisions, and it is here that the place of conflict becomes most clear. Four specific roles describe the manager as decision-maker: entrepreneur, disturbance handler, resource allocator and negotiator. As an entrepreneur, the manager seeks to improve the work unit, adapting it to changing environmental conditions.

Managers, concerned with growth and development, are on the lookout for good ideas, selectively developing them either personally or through the efforts of a subordinate. Because of scarce resources, not all good ideas can be pursued at a given time. Deciding from among options generates conflict as different members of the work group have vested interests in pursuing a particular course of action. Furthermore, as an entrepreneur, the manager becomes a voluntary initiator of change—a process fraught with conflict.

In contrast to the entrepreneur role where the manager initiates change, in the disturbance-handler role, the manager reacts to changes initiated outside his or her control. These situations may include a disciplinary problem, a staff shortage, etc. No manager can anticipate every contingency and every consequence of every action. The job of the manager in this respect has been likened to that of a conductor of a symphony orchestra. The conductor must try to perform a concert while the orchestra members are having various personal problems, the stage hands are moving equipment around and the temperature in the hall changes from hot to cold, creating discomfort for the audience and havoc for the instruments.

As an allocator of resources, the manager makes decisions that determine who gets what in the work group. Resources include personnel, the manager's time, money and equipment. In this role, the manager authorizes the important decisions of the unit before they are implemented, thus ensuring that decisions are interrelated. Unfortunately, the manager rarely has the time to consider the projects presented for approval in sufficient depth and at the optimal point in time. Two common solutions to this are to: (1) pick the proposer rather than the proposal, or

(2) put the decision off in the hope that it will go away.

In the first instance, projects are authorized whose sponsors are trusted. Such a process creates serious divisions among members of the work group as certain ones are correctly perceived as favorable regardless of the merits of their ideas. Avoiding decisions undermines the manager's power and effectiveness and often results in conflict among members of the work group because of the ambiguity resulting from unclear direction. What is avoided has the nasty habit of cropping up again and again, often entangled with other issues, making the decision process that much more complex.

Finally, the manager explicitly deals with conflict in negotiations: with other units, other professional groups, subordinates and hospital administrators for changes in policy and responsibilities, resolution of grievances, reallocation of resources and so forth. Such activities are common, if sometimes unpleasant. They are crucial to the work unit and to the manager's continued leadership role.

SOURCES OF CONFLICT

As the conflict inherent in each of the aforementioned roles is considered, a pattern emerges that is helpful in describing a finite number of major sources or categories of conflict. These sources include: hierarchical, interdepartmental, personnel system and interpersonal.

Hierarchical conflict

Hierarchical conflict results from the structure of the organization. As any system grows in complexity, it requires a division of labor and levels of management and authority through which work is coordinated toward a particular end. The health care organization is no different in this respect from other organizations. However, because it is predominantly a professional organization in which employees are educated and licensed outside the institution, problems of authority become exacerbated and expressed in hierarchical conflicts.

Challenges to the manager's authority by virtue of hierarchical position come in many forms. For the newly appointed supervisor, there is the testing of limits by subordinates, the indirect (and often the direct) lack of support for new ideas seen in less than timely and enthusiastic cooperation and the continuing undercurrent of dissatisfaction that someone else did not receive the promotion. Supervisors of professional staff tend to resist authority based on an erroneous assumption that professionals because they are paid and trained to exercise judgement, do not need supervision. This idea is directly related to the amount of autonomy the professional desires and how much is available in the position. Limited amounts of perceived available autonomy coupled with a fairly high degree of desired autonomy pave the way for conflict, as does the opposite condi-

tion. Clearly, there is a mismatch in the structure of the job, the opportunities available for individual initiative as dictated by the hierarchy or managerial style of superiors and the needs of the employee.

Interdepartmental conflict

Interdepartmental conflict is a frequent phenomenon in health care institutions as the values of one professional department clash with another. The most obvious case is the ongoing struggle between physicians and nurses. Whereas physicians and their values have dominated the health care delivery system, medical dominance has been challenged during the last decade, particularly by nurses and other health care providers as their roles and responsibilities have expanded.[2,3] The inevitable conflicts that arose as a result of one group wanting control and input into decisions once viewed as outside their legitimate domain have been a focal point for changes in levels of participation in health care institutions across the country.[4]

In a more general sense, interdepartmental conflict exists to some degree in all organizations. It becomes more pronounced in those where the reward structures are ambiguous and where the payoffs for collaborating across departmental lines are minimal or nonexistent. What is often perceived by supervisors is a zero-sum situation in which resources not geared to their immediate needs are regarded as general losses to the work group and as a gain to another group. This same reasoning is seen between individuals within a work unit and is the source of significant nonproductive conflict whereby a "we–they" mentality is fostered. Combating this orientation requires an emphasis on healthy competition within a framework of collaboration. At the base of such an orientation is the recognition that all departments, and for that matter all individuals within a department, are interdependent.

To survive, as well as thrive in the long run, requires some sacrifice of individual needs for departmental and organizational achievement. In turn, through departmental and organizational accomplishment, individual needs are furthered. One antidote to unit suboptimization, whereby each work group narrowly defines itself without consideration of its important linkages to others, is for the supervisor to articulate those linkages explicitly and to consider the impact of departmental activities on other departments. Soliciting input from people likely to be affected by proposed changes is an important step in reducing conflict brought about by turf issues. Although it is unreasonable to expect that all affected parties will support a particular change, bringing them into the decision process and seriously considering their concerns ultimately reduces conflict when implementation occurs.

Personnel system conflict

Conflict resulting from the personnel system occurs in relation to performance appraisal, discipline, benefits and compensation. At the heart of such conflict is, typically, a discrepancy in perceived equity whereby the treatment of one group or individual is seen as unfair relative to another. At an institutional level, for example, benefits and compensation for laboratory personnel may be regarded as inequitable relative to those at a comparable facility. Conflict will result to the extent that the employee feels unfairly treated. If the discrepancy cannot be resolved or understood and accepted (e.g., a temporary condition, offset by other factors) and the employee has work alternatives, resignation may result.

Where there are no alternatives and the perception of inequity continues, conflict and dissatisfaction will continue. Within a department, lack of clarity, arguments regarding performance goals and expectations, and failure to give timely feedback of a positive as well as of a constructively negative nature, will increase conflict and dissatisfaction with the appraisal process. Lack of consistency with regard to the exercise of discipline will be equally problematic.

Institutional policies—both formal and informal—can add to the difficulty. Where supervisors are required to justify above or below standard performance, the odds are that every-

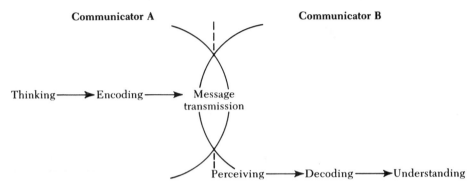

Figure 1. The communications process. Adapted with permission from Shannon, C.E., and Weaver, W. *The Mathematical Theory of Communication.* Urbana, IL: University of Illinois Press, 1949.

one in the department will receive standard ratings without sufficient regard to how well individuals perform. In the short run, this avoids conflict for the superior, who is not called upon to explain a rating. For superior performers, the process engenders frustration and conflict, often with the result of actually lowering their performance. The remedy requires that supervisors be expected to justify all performance reviews regardless of the rating. Although the supervisor may experience discomfort in anticipating a conflict situation with a disgruntled employee whose rating is below what the employee expected, when fairly applied and accompanied by adequate coaching, such a procedure can be most effective in reducing overall conflict and improving performance.

Interpersonal conflict

The area of interpersonal conflict has received the most significant attention in the literature on conflict in organizations. Although all of the conflict situations discussed so far ultimately involve interpersonal communication to clarify and resolve them, the source of the conflict lies outside the people involved in the interchange. Too often, this fact is ignored and the conflict is reduced to a fairly heated contest of wills. In the framework used here, the realm of interpersonal conflict includes communication and decision styles, both of which reflect personal values and needs.

Conflict resulting from communication styles emanates from the communications process itself. As seen in Figure 1, the traditional model of the process entails six basic components: thinking, encoding, transmission, perceiving, decoding and understanding. Thinking entails the sender framing the idea in his or her mind and associating the intent of the communication and the impact it should have on the receiver. The message (the idea and the interaction) is then encoded into a transmittable form. The form may be nonverbal, such as a greeting expressed in a handshake, or it may be expressed through writing or speech. The receiver must perceive that a message is being sent. The receiver then decodes the message by putting it in a form that renders it comprehensible. Finally, some meaning is assigned to the communication, which indicates understanding. Obviously, the goal of effective communication is to have the receiver interpret and understand the message as the sender intended.

The realities of organizational life suggest that breakdowns in interpersonal communications are a common event. Figure 2, demonstrating the dynamic feedback aspects of communications, provides some clues as to why breakdowns are so frequent and why conflict arises from them. Every interpersonal communication has a background or setting. For example, the performance appraisal interview and its ramifications set the stage for the interpersonal communications occurring within it. Add to this a dictatorial style on the part of the manager, a defensive posture on the part of the subordinate and a history of unpleasant exchanges between the participants, and the stage is set for multiple distortions in communications and subsequent conflict. The relationship between the communicators, the degree of trust, the use of authority, and expectations, all provide for context, as do the timing and locale of the interaction.

Breakdowns may occur even before transmission of the message. The sender's thoughts may be unclear, the interaction may not be conducive to an effective interaction (e.g., the sender is interested in one-upsmanship) or the encoding may be in terms that are unfamiliar to the receiver. The last is a frequent type of interpersonal conflict in which the sender uses professional jargon that is outside the receiver's field of experience. Although the intent behind the use of such jargon may be a power play, it frequently is the result of insensitivity to the receiver's experience. Because of the diversity of professional groups working within the health care setting, communications between members of different groups have a higher chance of breaking down because of inaccurate assumptions concerning shared language.

Because of the diversity of professional groups working within the health care setting, communications between members of different groups have a higher chance of breaking down.

The lack of shared meaning, the lack of specificity and clarity in the message and the tendency to treat assumptions as though they were facts create much conflict in communications.

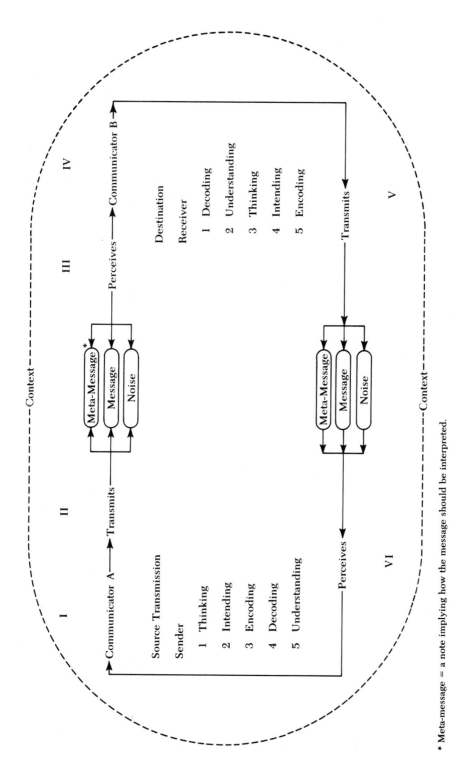

* Meta-message = a note implying how the message should be interpreted.

Figure 2. The feedback or double-loop communications model. Reprinted with permission from Numerof, R.E. *The Practice of Management for Health Care Professionals*. New York: American Management Association, 1982, p. 302.

Problems in transmission also create communications conflict, mainly through the interference of "noise." Noise may come in many forms, including distractions and impatience that either the sender or receiver brings to the situation and distractions in the physical surroundings (e.g., telephones and beepers interrupting meetings, people walking in and out of meetings).

Finally, the ability for clear, concise and congruent self-expression greatly influences the degree to which conflict will occur in communications, and when it does occur, to what extent it will be managed effectively.[5] Styles that are passive–aggressive, or indirect in the expression of needs and opinions, particularly disagreement and conflict, create additional conflict. Similarly, an aggressive style that dominates interpersonal interaction without due consideration for the values and opinions of others exacerbates conflict and sets the stage for a passive–aggressive response.

COMMUNICATIONS STYLES

Passive–aggressive style

Passive–aggressive communication is intended to hide anger and avoid conflict. The passive–aggressive communicator denies his or her feelings, avoids taking risks and tries to stay out of trouble by not "hurting" others. The intended gain is to win the approval of others, be liked or express hostility indirectly when direct expression is perceived to be dangerous. The nonverbal communications that accompany this style include downcast eyes (thus avoiding direct eye contact); soft, barely audible voice and hesitation in speech; helpless gestures; and slumped posture. Verbally, this type of communication denies or minimizes the importance of the situation, conveys the message that "anything you want is okay with me," or avoids the situation altogether. The receiver of such communication usually does not respond as the passive–aggressive individual desires.

Passive–aggressive behavior is generally interpreted by others as suggesting that the sender does not know what he or she is talking about, is a pushover, has little conviction in his or her own ideas or is uncooperative and obstructive. These interpretations result in others taking advantage of or manipulating the passive–aggressive person, making unreasonable requests, denying legitimate requests, and generally being disrespectful and disagreeable. Passive–aggressive responses to such treatment include manipulation, withdrawal, noncompliance or compliance to the other person in the situation. These responses engender considerable anger in the recipients of the behavior, whose responses (e.g., outrage) often ignite further passive–aggressive behavior and unresolved conflict. In an organizational culture where the norms dictate "stay in your place," "don't make waves" and submit to others, particularly in relation to those higher in the organization, the stage is set for passive–aggressive, dysfunctional communication and conflict.

There are also a number of personally held destructive attitudes that promote indirect communications. These include the following:
- Getting angry is destructive and a waste of time.
- If I say how I really feel, he or she will not be able to handle it and will fall apart, be hurt or in some way be damaged.
- If I let go of my angry feelings, I may lose control over myself.
- Being direct is inappropriate behavior.
- If I'm open about my feelings, others will reject me.
- I'm afraid of what others will do to retaliate.
- Other people's needs and feelings are much more important than mine.
- It is easier to say yes than to deal with the guilt of refusing someone's request.

Aggressive style

At the other end of the spectrum from passive–aggressive communications style lies aggressive communications style. It has as its hallmark a lack of fear in the direct expression of needs, opinions and feelings, coupled with a lack of concern about others' needs, opinions and feelings. Aggressive communications is intended to be self-expressive and dominant, with an underlying goal of "setting

others straight." The aggressive communicator believes that communications is a win–lose proposition. Thus to gain one's goals entails a loss. Compromise is also equated with loss. The nonverbal communications that accompany this style include glaring and piercing eye contact, loud voice, fluent and fast speech, threatening gestures, intimidating postures and confrontation.

The receiver of such communication usually interprets the behavior as being rude and thoughtless, and intended to be hurtful. The aggressive communicator may be seen as pompous and without feelings. If the participants in a communication exchange are equal in status and power, the response may be counteraggression (i.e., hostile remarks, loud voice or threats) and escalating conflict. Typically, however, and particularly where there is status inequality as in the case of status differentials across professional or hierarchical lines, the stage is set for passive–aggressive responses and unresolved conflict.

Directed style

The communications style most likely to resolve conflict effectively as it arises is the directed style. It entails communications techniques that minimize distortion and increase the probability that a given individual's needs will be met without resulting in loss for others. The assumptions in directed communications include:
- that individuals have the right to their own feelings, thoughts and ideas;

- that individuals have the right and freedom to express these as long as they do not impinge on others' rights to their own feelings, thoughts and ideas; and
- that individuals have responsibility for their own feelings and must acquire respect for those of others.[6]

Directed communications style places the expression of personal ideas and opinions in a social context. People in organizations must assume responsibility for their feelings and ideas and display sensitivity for the possible effect that they may have on receivers. Freedom of self-expression is not license to say whatever one wants with impunity. The essence of this approach is to take responsibility in communications by using "I messages" without hinting, using sarcasm or intentionally hurting or embarrassing the receiver. Eye contact is direct, speech is fluent and firm, and responses are in direct response to the situation. The receiver of such communication is likely to perceive that the sender is confident and honest, conveying both self-respect and respect for the recipient.

One model the author has used in organizations throughout the country has demonstrated excellent results in minimizing communication distortions and thus reducing and resolving conflict. It is called the Description, Expression, Specification and Consequences (DESC) Model and is based on a four-step communication sequence.

The DESC Model, because it is sit-uation neutral, can be applied in any type of conflict situation with promising results. The following case illustrates its use in intervention in an ongoing conflict with elements from three of the four sources of conflict described previously (i.e., hierarchical, interdepartmental and interpersonal). Although, for conceptual purposes, various sources of conflict can be clearly delineated, in reality these sources overlap, making conflict and its resolution more complex. The overlapping aspect is illustrated in the following case, and the DESC Model is then applied in resolving it.

A CASE IN POINT

Good Samaritan Hospital, a 600-bed facility located in a large eastern metropolitan city, is a nonprofit institution with a commitment to staff development and training as a way of improving patient care, productivity and staff morale. There has been increased interest on the part of senior administration to consult with the education department to further this end.

The director of education, FR, met the challenge with mixed feelings, none of which were shared with her administrative superior. She was afraid of appearing less than competent in her role. As she saw it, her staff were being asked to move in new directions without clear administrative support, without the necessary technical skills to facilitate the transition and without enthusiasm from potential recipients of the new services. The last aspect was particularly troublesome as one of her supervisors had noted resistance to the department's involvement with nursing services and the laboratory. The most recent incident involved the laboratory.

HB, an education supervisor, had been requested to revise a training program that his department had prepared previously for the laboratory. To date, this program had been run over a four-week time span and focused on the technical and quality control aspects of laboratory work. One criticism of the program was its failure to provide follow through to assess the extent to which participants incorporated the information in their work. The laboratory's criticism had not been shared with HB or his colleagues. However, no one from the education department had specifically solicited constructive criticism regarding the training efforts. Because attendance at the programs was good, HB assumed all was well.

In recognition of the importance of inservice education in this and related areas, the laboratory department hired a full-time staff member to assume technical training. The position was a new one and would allow for some creativity in its development.

FR was under the impression that her department and SP, a laboratory specialist hired to assume technical training, would be working collaboratively in the redesign of the course in question as well as in the design of future courses. Quite to her surprise,

SP undertook complete responsibility for the course, and HB was relegated to an assisting role under SP's supervision. Given HB's more senior status as a supervisor, this was extremely hard for him to accept.

HB presented a detailed and fairly lengthy proposal to outline the redesign of the course, which incorporated both didactic material and clinical evaluation. The proposal was rejected by the laboratory, primarily because of the suggested time frame. Although it proposed offering the course quarterly, the department wanted it available on a more frequent basis, particularly since it was used as an orientation course for new employees. Given that turnover occurred fairly frequently, the laboratory department wanted it available on a regular basis. HB reworked the proposal and resubmitted it with a new timetable. The revised proposal was rejected, as were subsequent attempts to work with the laboratory department in collaborative development of new courses. FR heard via the managerial grapevine that HB was abrasive and uncooperative.

This case clearly demonstrates a number of serious conflicts common in organizations. The question of interdepartmental turf is most obvious in terms of control over educational programs in the institution. There is a lack of clarity regarding the goals and responsibilities of the education department vis-à-vis the laboratory, particularly as they relate to "internal consultation." A nondirect communications style adopted by the director of education fails to clarify with administration what the Department of Education's new role entails and what supports would be required for it to succeed.

Another serious avoidance was the failure to confront the potential undermining of the education department by the hiring of the laboratory specialist who reported only to the director of the laboratory. These avoidances reflect discomfort on the part of the education director in handling conflict within the hierarchy—this time in relation to her superior. Hierarchical conflict was also demonstrated with the education supervisor's discomfort in playing a facilitative role to someone who, although did not directly report to her, was lower in positional status. The end result was a common and unfortunate one. Namely, the problem was defined as an interpersonal one, and a single employee was identified as the problem. In this case and in many similar situations, the problem was many faceted and longstanding. It began with problems in clarity of roles, goals and procedures, and was exacerbated by indirect communications styles on the part of numerous participants.

A helpful intervention would be for FR to call a meeting with the laboratory director to clarify roles and responsibilities. Using the DESC model, she might approach the situation as follows:

- Description: "It has come to my attention that a number of recent attempts for collaboration be-

tween your department and mine have not worked. The ones I am thinking of have involved the work of HB and SP on the technical course."
- Expression: "I am concerned about the failure to come to a mutual agreement and the bad feelings that seem to have resulted."
- Specification: "I would like to meet with you this week to discuss the situation and better understand what went wrong."
- Consequences: "I think that clarifying this situation and our respective roles and responsibilities will resolve any bad feelings that may remain between the departments and pave the way to better collaboration between us in the future."

The stage is now set for a productive, nondefensive meeting and a future working relationship in which conflict is confronted directly.

IMPLICATIONS FOR THE MANAGER

The health care environment is a stressful environment because of the nature of the work, which often involves matters of life and death. The complexity of health and medical care requires that many people need to work closely together. Interdependence, particularly where there are limited resources, inevitably leads to conflict. Add to this a status hierarchy not shared by all, differing values, questionable trust and stereotyped perceptions and the amount of conflict will be increased. The manager as conflict negotiator must be able to deal with his or her own expression of conflict. The manager must also be able to surface underlying disagreements and develop norms in the work group that promote: (1) the expression of difference with respect and tolerance for alternative positions and (2) the constructive criticism of ideas without attacking the promoters of those ideas. Cognizant of the pervasiveness of conflict, alert to the dangers of mismanaged and ignored conflict and armed with a model to manage it effectively, the supervisor increases his or her effectiveness as a manager.

REFERENCES

1. Mintzberg, H. *The Structuring of Organizations.* Englewood Cliffs, N.J.: Prentice-Hall, 1979.
2. Freidson, E. *Professional Dominance: The Social Structure of Medical Care.* New York: Atherton Press, 1970.
3. Numerof, R.E. *The Practice of Management for Health Care Professionals.* New York: AMACOM, 1982.
4. National Commission on Nursing. Initial Report and Preliminary Recommendations. Chicago: American Hospital Association, 1981.
5. Numerof, R.E. *Managing Stress: A Guide for Health Professionals.* Rockville, MD: Aspen Systems, 1983.
6. Numerof, *Managing Stress.*

Absenteeism: A nurse manager's concern

Kip DeWeese
Head Nurse
Rehabilitation
McKay-Dee Hospital Center
Ogden, Utah

ABSENTEEISM is a managerial problem for many work organizations today. Nurse managers and administrators should be concerned with this problem. Workable solutions could be in place to help combat absenteeism, or solutions could be quickly adapted to help reduce the extent of its impact. Before looking at such measures as staff recruitment, bonuses, or bringing in unskilled labor, however, nurse managers might do well to study all dimensions of the problem of nursing absenteeism.

In hospitals, it appears that nursing absenteeism is continually placing a strain on already scarce resources. This strain is evident not only in economic terms but in organizational effectiveness as well. Factors that are manifest in this problem are: (1) the costs for replacement of absent individuals; (2) the resultant loss of productivity; and (3) inferior quality nursing care for clients. These elements

Health Care Superv, 1987, 5(3), 69–76
© 1987 Aspen Publishers, Inc.

have significance when it is considered that in most hospitals 90 percent of absent nurses require replacement, often at overtime rates of pay.[1]

Schneller examines the numerous costs associated with absenteeism. There are the direct salary costs of increased overtime or overstaffing necessary to perform the duties of absent workers. Fringe benefit expenses that the absent worker continues to receive (e.g., insurance, pension, vacation, holiday) add up quickly. Costs of maintaining and administering an absence control program, whether effective or not, might be important considerations. There are several indirect and hard-to-measure costs.

(a) increased supervisory time spent revising work schedules, counseling and reprimanding workers, and checking the work quality of substitutes; (b) lowered morale among workers who may resent doing someone else's work and a consequent higher level of turnover, grievances, and tardiness; and (c) reduced productivity from more work being done by people who are less experienced and/or fatigued.[2]

Factors such as these are much more evident today because the number of short-term absences is rising, with a smaller component of sickness and longer absences. Kleinman writes that "studies done over the past few years have revealed the duration of absence has been decreasing but the frequency of spells has been increasing."[3]

While addressing the issue of absenteeism at a meeting at General Motors Corporation a number of years ago, James M. Roche gave a graphic description of the implications of having workers absent from their stations.

We've got absenteeism in our plants, which is common throughout the industry, running twice as high as it did a few years ago, etc. You can't run a business on this basis, effectively or efficiently, because the highest days in the week for absenteeism are Fridays and Mondays. So absenteeism of 13–15 percent is fairly common. Well, when you get ready to start an assembly line and you find out that you have 13 percent of the people gone, you have to do a lot of scrounging. You have to bring people over to try to man the stations, who are not proficient or who have not had the experience. You've got to double your supervision, you've got to double your inspection and this creates an insurmountable burden.[4]

Simply defined, absenteeism is the failure of the worker to appear on the job when scheduled to work. This can be time lost because of illness or because of accident. It can be unauthorized time away from the job. Any person who is absent from work is referred to as an absentee.[5]

In analyzing the problem of absenteeism it is the unscheduled absences and the chronic absences that the nurse manager should be most concerned with.

UNSCHEDULED ABSENCES

Unscheduled absences are absences by staff members that occur outside of the legitimate use of their allotted sick days. This type of absence occurs when the reason for the absence is not valid or cannot be attributed to illness or to any other emergency. Here one must keep in mind

that the word "sickness" may have little value, particularly when related to short-term uncertificated spells of absence. There is no realistic way to determine the sickness component of any period of absence. Essentially, the decision not to go to work lies with the individual, and the reasons given by the employee for short spells of absence may be fictitious.[6]

A worker who averages one or more days per week or four or more days per month for two successive months without a valid reason is considered to be a chronic absentee.

CHRONIC ABSENCE

Chronic absence occurs when a person has made it a habit to be absent, whether the absences are valid or invalid. "A worker who averages one or more days per week or four or more days per month for two successive months without a valid reason is considered to be a chronic absentee."[7] Chronic absenteeism can pose other considerations for the nurse manager. McDonald describes different types of chronic absentees. For the nurse manager to deal with them, he has written

occasionally . . . no matter how hard the nursing supervisor has tried to set an example by personal, regular attendance, patiently listened to excuses, repeatedly explained policies, and even "off-the-record" discussed the employee's attendance as a well intentioned counselor or friend, that supervisor will run into a severe case of chronic "absenteeitis." In dealing with the chronic absentee, the nursing supervisor must not be swayed by repeated excuses.[8]

Hypochondria

The first type of chronic absentee discussed by McDonald is the hypochondriac absentee. This employee will use maximum sick leave, complain of aches and pains while at work, and attempt to sway supervisors to feel sympathetic when returning to work. To deal with this the nurse manager should try to avoid discussing symptoms, but calmly point out to the hypochondriac the problems that this behavior is causing the rest of the nursing team and the manager.

Immaturity

Another type of chronic absenteeism is exhibited by the immature absentee. This person is not necessarily young in years, but is, however, likely to lack the self-discipline that normally comes with adulthood. The immature absentee probably does not have any pressing financial responsibilities and therefore does not feel especially anxious about losing employment. This absentee is restless and easily influenced by other nursing staff who also may take time off. The nurse manager, through careful questioning, may even find that this person actually believes that management expects occasional absence from everyone.

For the nurse manager, then, this is a case of trying to straighten out the youngster by assuming a parent role and teaching the employee more effective work habits.

Escapism

The escapist absentee stays away from work because of boredom with the job and typically does not think about the long-term consequences of this type of behavior. This absentee also is probably impulsive and unwilling to postpone the gratification of a delayed day off or future vacation. The nurse manager needs to try to identify the reason for work boredom, such as person–job mismatch, and needs patience and counseling skills to turn the escapist around.

Abusiveness

The abusive absentee can be extremely difficult to deal with. This person probably is taking time off to get back at the nursing management team for some real or, more likely, imagined wrongdoing on the part of a particular nurse manager or fellow employee. The excuse "If Joe can get away with it then so can I" will be offered when the abusive absentee is confronted by the nurse manager, and the employee is likely to be hostile and resentful during confronta-

tion. This person will often challenge the nurse manager's right to use disciplinary action.

Poor motivation

The poorly motivated absentee is also a chronic absentee and is one who sees the job simply as a paycheck. This employee will often not participate in unit affairs and seldom does more than the minimum required to keep from getting fired. To deal with this person the manager needs to look at motivation and possibly gear counseling to focus on "What is in it for the employee," appeal to the employee's sense of self-respect and pride, and help the person see how it is possible to contribute to the team.

The final type of chronic absentee is the "burned-out absentee" who was once a highly motivated, dedicated staff member but has lost enthusiasm and zeal for the job of providing care. The real problem here is psychological, and often a skilled and understanding counselor who works well with the burnout syndrome can help restore this person to his or her former well-praised level of functioning.[9]

FACTORS CONTRIBUTING TO ABSENTEEISM

Factors that contribute to the overall problem of absenteeism also are important for the nurse manager to understand. Generally, these factors can be grouped under three major titles: external, or extrinsic, causes; internal, or intrinsic, causes; and personality causes.

External and internal causes

External causes may include such things as weather conditions or distance to travel to get to work. Extrinsic causes may be fostered by such factors as liberal personnel policies, lack of attendance policies, lack of communication, lack of effective employee selection, or low pay and unpleasant working conditions.[10] Internal or intrinsic causes are factors such as job boredom, ineffective supervision, poor inter- or intragroup work relations, lack of control in making decisions affecting one's work, and over-work and physical exhaustion.[11] While it is easy to label these causes as "lack of motivation" or "improper attitude," as McDonald and Shaver mention, "To do so is to overlook the influence management can and does have over them."[12] In other words, management can, perhaps, do something about them.

Personality causes

Personality causes, on the other hand, are more challenging for the nurse manager to deal with, because it is difficult for the nurse manager to change behavior. Such change must of course come from the individual employee. However, again as McDonald and Shaver point out, "An effective administrator can exercise some control over personality related

absences."[13] Characteristic of personality absences are such signs as personality conflicts, the absence-prone personality, problems related to drug and alcohol abuse, family problems, and illness. Here it is interesting to note, as does Rowland, some demographic factors related to family problems. "Female workers have a higher absolute absenteeism rate and it is rising faster than that of males. Age is inversely related to absenteeism; the highest rates are in the 18–25 year old age group and the lowest in the 40–65 group. Both unmarried males and females have a lower absenteeism rate than the married group."[14]

A word of caution to those concerned about personal absence: Although personality absences do figure into the total absence picture, some personal absences are absolutely necessary for the employee who has experienced some type of personal trauma (e.g., death of a spouse or parent, or divorce); the person needs time off to restore personal equilibrium.[15]

DEALING WITH ABSENTEEISM

While it is helpful to understand absenteeism, the type of absences, and the causes of absences, where can one actually start in order to deal effectively with the problem? The first step is to actually document that the problem exists. As Harris writes "obtaining easily understandable information is the key to decision making."[16] He then lists a step-by-step method whereby the nurse manager can easily identify and document an absentee problem.

Documenting the problem

First, the average of full-time employees assigned to the department is needed. Counting the employees at the beginning and end of any month and averaging provides a mid-month number of employees. Or even simpler, the number of full-time equivalents (FTEs) of a department can be used.

Second, this work force (either FTEs or mid-month number of employees) is multiplied by a constant number of days scheduled per employee per month. This number can be computed by subtracting the number of vacation, holiday, etc., days allowed by the institution from the number of theoretical days an employee can work annually.

For example, assuming an employee is scheduled to work 5 days per week for 52 weeks, the maximum number of days the employee could work annually would be 260. By subtracting 10 vacation days, 8 holidays, and 2 other benefit days, the employee will work 240 days per year, or 20 days per month. This constant, 20 days per month, is then multiplied by the average number of employees assigned, thus equaling the total number of days scheduled per month for a department.[17]

The third step is to figure the number of unplanned absences during the month by simply keeping track of who is absent and when.[18]

The fourth step is to compute the absence rate. The method most frequently used and recommended by the Bureau of Employment Security of the U.S. Department of Labor is:

$$\frac{\text{Absentee}}{\text{rate}} = \frac{\begin{array}{c}\text{Total days lost}\\\text{due to absence}\end{array} \times 100}{\text{Total days scheduled}}[19]$$

According to figures released by the Bureau of National Affairs (BNA) that state that nine or more absences per year constitute unsatisfactory attendance, an absentee rate of three to five percent annually can be considered poor employee performance.[20]

This four-step tool presented by Harris can be used by the nurse manager to examine the problem of absenteeism at any level—institutional, departmental, or individual employee. This tool also does not require computer assistance, and it definitely helps managers and employees see the problem. As Harris writes: "Becoming aware of an absentee problem and letting the employee know that management is aware of the problem is part of providing leadership to the group and to the individual."[21] This is all that may be needed to show an immediate improvement in the problem of absenteeism.

Evaluating sick leave plans

Literature suggests that nurse managers should evaluate sick leave plans afforded by their organizations, because liberal sick leave plans and policies actually lend themselves to

Literature suggests that liberal sick leave plans and policies actually lend themselves to higher rates of absenteeism.

higher rates of absenteeism.[22] Rowland suggests a basic solution with sick leave plans called "checkup and surveillance." With this method the absentee with a one-day sickness excuse is sent, upon return, to the employee health clinic to explain the causes or symptoms to the physician. A variation of this method is to have a nurse, hired for this purpose, actually visit absentee workers' homes to find out how they feel or determine if medical help is needed. This solicitude fools no one, nor is it meant to. In one hospital, however, substantial reductions in sick leave time have been achieved since the method was instituted.[23]

Another answer to poor sick leave programs is a combined program in which all leave—vacation, sick days, and holidays—is paid to the employee from one account that is earned according to hours and days worked.[24] A similar program, outlined by Cwiek, is an earned-time policy, wherein the benefits accrue according to hours and days worked. There is, however, a probationary period, in which the employee can take no paid leave time. After probation, an employee can draw sick leave only if he or she is hospitalized or misses three consecutive days from work because of illness.[25]

Besides working in conjunction with other organizational administrators in developing and adopting a workable sick leave plan, and in addition to confronting an employee with documented evidence of an absenteeism problem, the nurse manager could also do well to apply a progressive discipline attendance policy. The nurse manager probably will find that some form of discipline regarding absenteeism is essential, and such a system imposes increasingly severe penalties on unexcused, or in some cases, even excused absences. "The basis of such a policy is that employees know in advance what the consequences of their behavior will be."[26] In determining the type of discipline, it is important to keep in mind that legal risks may arise; therefore, it is essential that such policies be consistent, fair, and carefully documented.

• • •

Nurse absenteeism can be either a hidden or a visible problem that nurse managers should deal with. In today's immediate challenges to nursing administration, decreasing absenteeism and bringing it into line could be a means toward dramatic savings to the institution, and most assuredly, it would have much to do with maintaining the quality of client care.

REFERENCES

1. Kleinman, J., and Rosberger, Z. "Stringing Phenomena: Analysis of Nursing Absenteeism." *Hospital and Health Services Administration* 27, no. 6 (1982): 59.
2. Schneller, G.O., Kopelman, R.E., and Silver, J.J. "A Combined Leave Benefit System for the Control of Absenteeism in Health Care Organizations." *Hospital and Health Services Administration* 27, no. 1 (1982): 64.
3. Kleinman and Rosberger, "Stringing Phenomena: Analysis of Nursing Absenteeism," 60.
4. Hartman, R.I., and Gibson, J.J. "The Persistent Problem of Employee Absenteeism." *Personnel Journal* 50, no. 7 (1971): 535.
5. Felt, B.L. "Absenteeism in Nursing." *Nursing Management* 13, no. 1 (1982): 35–38.
6. Kleinman and Rosberger, "Stringing Phenomena: Analysis of Nursing Absenteeism," 62.
7. Ibid., 35.
8. McDonald, J.M., and Shaver, A.V. "An Absenteeism Control Program." *Journal of Nursing Administration* 11, no. 5 (1981): 13–18.
9. Ibid., 17–18.
10. Ibid., 13.
11. Ibid., 13.
12. Ibid., 13.
13. Ibid., 14
14. Rowland, H.S., and Rowland, B.L. *Nursing Administration Handbook.* Rockville, Md.: Aspen Publishers, 1981, pp. 295–305.
15. Felt, "Absenteeism in Nursing," 36.
16. Harris, H.O. "A Practical Approach to an Absenteeism Program." *Hospital Topics* 59, no. 2 (1981): 15–17.
17. Ibid., 15–16.
18. McDonald and Shaver, "An Absenteeism Control Program," 16.
19. Harris, "A Practical Approach to an Absenteeism Program," 16.
20. McDonald and Shaver, "An Absenteeism Control Program," 16.
21. Harris, "A Practical Approach to an Absenteeism Program," 17.
22. Schneller, Kopelman, and Silver, "A Combined Leave Benefit System for the Control of Absenteeism in Health Care Organizations," 64.
23. Rowland and Rowland, *Nursing Administration Handbook*, 298.
24. Schneller, Kopelman, and Silver, "A Combined Leave Benefit System for the Control of Absenteeism in Health Care Organizations," 64.
25. Cwiek, M.A. "Earned Time Policy Aims to Improve RN Attendance." *Hospital Progress* 63, no. 2 (1982): 49–50.
26. McDonald and Shaver, "An Absenteeism Control Program," 17.

How to delegate effectively

Carol A. Distasio
President
D&E Health Educational Systems,
  Inc.
Baltimore, Maryland

JOHN is the medical director of a busy adolescent clinic in an inner-city neighborhood. He has asked his secretary, Sara, to open, screen and route the mail that comes into the clinic. Sara seldom gets to do this, because if John happens to pass by her desk when the mail arrives, he picks up the entire bundle, takes it into his office and sorts through it himself. It is not unusual for John to put some of the mail into his "for home" briefcase, some on his desk (which is continually cluttered) and some back on Sara's desk. Lately some of the mail has been getting lost after it arrives in the pediatric clinic. Tempers are beginning to flare over problems related to how the mail is handled. Sara is frustrated because she feels she has no control over the mail. She has asked the clinic director not to remove the mail before she has had an opportunity to screen and distribute it, but he continues to do so anyway.

Health Care Superv, 1985,3(4),67–80
© 1985 Aspen Publishers, Inc.

Louellen is a nursing supervisor in charge of five busy medical-surgical units. She believes strongly in delegation and routinely issues directives to all levels of subordinate nursing service personnel as she makes clinical rounds from unit to unit. Yesterday Louellen told a nursing assistant on Hall 1 to have the linen closet straightened by 11:00 A.M., instructed a licensed practical nurse on Hall 3 to inventory intravenous supplies by 1:00 P.M. and directed the head nurse on Hall 5 to update all nursing care plans by 2:00 P.M. Staff on all three units were angered and resentful but they tried to comply with her directives.

When Louellen returned to check on whether these tasks had been accomplished, she found that none had been done. She chastised certain employees, although they attempted to make her aware of patient care problems and other unit conditions and circumstances that prevented them from accomplishing the tasks within the time frame Louellen had specified. Louellen responded by telling staff that they did not know how to manage their time and that she expected them to improve their job performance in the future. Staff members were increasingly hostile and exhibited avoidance behaviors when Louellen made her last rounds. A review of time and attendance, absenteeism and turnover on Louellen's units indicates that her personnel have consistently higher rates of all these variables than personnel in other clinical units.

CASE ANALYSIS

What is wrong in these situations? John has delegated an appropriate task to an appropriate subordinate, but he repeatedly interferes with the delegatee's task accomplishment. Worse, he is unaware of the effects of his behavior on his secretary and other staff and on unit operations. Although his secretary has discussed this issue with him, his behavior continues unchanged. This situation clearly illustrates not only problems with delegation, but supervisory problems relating to time management, interpersonal relations and the general management of day-to-day unit operations.

What about Louellen's case? According to policies and procedures at Louellen's hospital, she has delegated appropriate tasks to appropriate personnel. However, Louellen's pattern of delegation is incorrect: she delegated without being fully aware of changing conditions on the units, did not inquire about shifting priorities, established arbitrary time limits that staff were unable to meet, demonstrated insensitivity to patient care priorities and staff concerns, and reprimanded and intimidated staff when they tried to explain why delegated tasks had not been accomplished as assigned. These managerial behaviors predictably resulted in more time and attendance problems and higher absenteeism and turnover rates among personnel in the units under Louellen's supervisory jurisdiction.

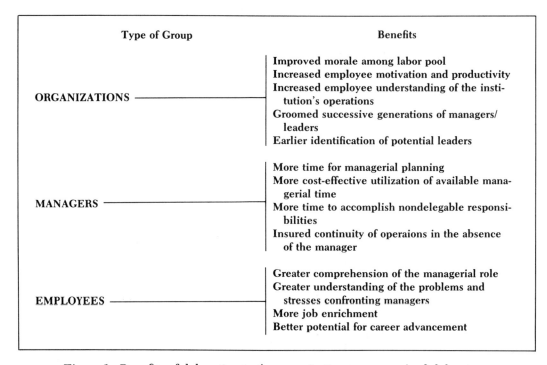

Type of Group	Benefits
ORGANIZATIONS	Improved morale among labor pool Increased employee motivation and productivity Increased employee understanding of the institution's operations Groomed successive generations of managers/leaders Earlier identification of potential leaders
MANAGERS	More time for managerial planning More cost-effective utilization of available managerial time More time to accomplish nondelegable responsibilities Insured continuity of operaions in the absence of the manager
EMPLOYEES	Greater comprehension of the managerial role Greater understanding of the problems and stresses confronting managers More job enrichment Better potential for career advancement

Figure 1. Benefits of delegation to the organization, managers and delegatees.

WHY DELEGATE?

How delegation, when done correctly, benefits organizations, managers and employees is illustrated in Figure 1. Effective delegation frees managerial time for other tasks that cannot be delegated, such as planning, and for those managerial functions that require special expertise, experience, knowledge or creativity and thus cannot be delegated.[1,2]

Delegation provides subordinates with the opportunity to expand their job capabilities, enrich their day-to-day work experience, increase their self-esteem and enhance their career potential. Delegatees develop a greater comprehension of manage-

ment functions and are better prepared to assume components of the managerial role in the manager's absence. Further, employees who perform delegated tasks well tend to demonstrate increased motivation and productivity as well as increased interest in the organization in general.

From an organizational perspective, delegation also helps assure that

---

Employees who perform delegated tasks well tend to demonstrate increased motivation and productivity as well as increased interest in the organization in general.

---

potential managers are constantly being groomed for career advancement. Further, subordinates who have been delegated some aspects of the managerial role will have had some experience in managing should it become necessary for them to function in an acting administrative position.[3-5]

DELEGATOR PREREQUISITES

To delegate effectively, managers must recognize the benefits of delegating and feel comfortable relinquishing some of the managerial role. Not only must they be willing to delegate, but they must have the temperament and the wisdom to provide the delegatee with appropriate managerial supports while encouraging and permitting the delegatee to accomplish the assigned task autonomously. Managers must accept the fact that, though a delegatee may not perform a delegated task in the same way that the manager would have done it, as long as the task is accomplished satisfactorily and on time the delegating has been successful.

IDENTIFYING TASKS THAT CAN BE DELEGATED

Tasks that are routine and that do not require special expertise or a high level of individual creativity should automatically be delegated. In contrast, tasks that require particular expertise or experience, are highly technical in nature or involve long-range planning for departments or units should not be delegated. Hir-

ing, firing, personnel policy formulation and developing reorganization strategies are managerial responsibilities that cannot normally be delegated.

Consider the following situation. Henry is the recently appointed director of operations for a 400-bed long-term care facility. He retired from the military and this position is a second career for him. The organization is progressive and seeks to expand its operations. Henry has been asked to formulate a plan that would permit expansion by establishing additional facilities. These additional facilities would be senior citizen apartments, and residents would have a continuum of health care available within the same health care organization should nursing home placement become necessary as they age. Henry's boss Robert, the vice president of operations, has instructed Henry to include the following components in the expansion plan: budget, time schedule, bid procedures, staffing, facility size, resident eligibility guidelines and potential sites. New to his position, Henry delegates the drafting of the initial expansion proposal to Mary, his administrative assistant, a woman who has been employed at the facility for 15 years. As he directs her to write the draft he jokingly states, "You've been around here long enough to know what will fly!" The administrative assistant feels overwhelmed by her new superior's expectations, the nature of the project he has delegated to her and the fact that he will not only hold her accountable for formulating the initial draft for future facility development but will also expect her work to satisfy his expectations.

Mary quickly becomes distraught over the assignment. One evening she encounters Robert as she is leaving work. She has known him for 12 years, their families attend the same church and their children have attended the same schools. In fact, at one time Mary was Robert's secretary. Robert, who is Henry's immediate supervisor, notices that Mary seems distressed. He asks her how things are going with her new boss. Frazzled, Mary blurts out her concerns and anxieties over the assignment Henry has delegated to her. Robert immediately recognizes the inappropriateness of delegating the task, the fact that Mary is not qualified to perform the task, and the unnecessary stress the assignment is provoking in a valued employee who has considerable longevity in the system. Robert, who has advanced to his current position through the ranks, directs Mary to stop working on the assignment, informs her that he will talk with Henry in the morning, and asks her to keep him informed should any other problems of this nature arise. When Henry arrives at his office the next morning, he is told to report immediately to Robert's office. Henry emerges from Robert's office 45 minutes later chagrined and chastised. He had been completely unaware of the problems his assignment created, and he was astounded to learn that his subordinate had discussed the assignment with his immediate superior.

What went wrong? Clearly, delegating the task was wholly inappropriate: if the administrative assistant could design a competent proposal for facility expansion, Henry (who was earning much higher wages) was certainly not needed to perform this task. But more was wrong than simply inappropriately delegating a task to an unqualified employee. Henry recently emerged from a military career. He was used to an autocratic system in which subordinates did not question orders. He was also insensitive to the informal corporate culture and informal power structure within his new work setting: his boss and his administrative assistant both had longevity in the system; they had worked together harmoniously in the past, continued to communicate in the workplace and had multiple religious, school and neighborhood linkages that complemented the work place linkages. Henry's behavior demonstrated his naiveté about the civilian system. Worse, it indicated that he had failed to thoroughly assess his new occupational situation and the major formal and informal system variables that could influence his position. Further, his behavior in this instance demonstrated a rather startling insensitivity to gender-related work place issues (e.g., comparable worth, gender-linked pay differences) and a cavalier attitude toward female subordinates.

The situation is interesting. Unless Henry is able to modify his attitudes and behaviors to accommodate his new work place environment, he might not survive in the system. From a management perspective this is as it should be; it would be cost and time inefficient to retain a manager exhibiting counterproductive behaviors—in this case, overdelegation.

PROBLEMS WITH DELEGATION

Problems with delegation arise for many reasons. Some are caused by managerial behaviors and some by delegatee responses. When problems arise with delegation, it is important to assess all aspects of the delegation process, identify the cause of the problems and plan effective managerial interventions to eliminate repeated failures.

Problems may also be caused by underdelegation and overdelegation. Overdelegation occurs when tasks are delegated to employees who are not qualified to perform them successfully. In such instances, delegatees exhibit various behaviors as they attempt to accomplish the delegated tasks:

- increased frustration, anger and discouragement as they continue to fail to achieve goals;
- repeated, but inadequate, efforts to get the task done;
- diminished self-esteem; and
- increased anxiety and apprehension as they continue to fall short of their goals.

Underdelegation occurs when tasks are assigned to persons who are overqualified to perform them. For ex-

Underdelegation occurs when tasks are assigned to persons who are overqualified to perform them.

ample, a professor at one of the local colleges has assigned one of her graduate students to a hospital as part of the student's administrative field experience. At the hospital the graduate student is placed in the president's office and directed to assist the president's executive aide with office correspondence, including typing, photocopying and filing. The student, whose family is making many financial sacrifices to help him obtain an advanced degree, attempts repeatedly to talk with hospital administration about being given a more appropriate administrative assignment. His efforts fail because the hospital president views graduate students as free clerical help. Two weeks after being assigned, the graduate student complains to his college professor, provides documentation that the field experience is not appropriate to course content or degree preparation and is reassigned to another health care institution.

Managerial behaviors that prevent successful delegation

Some managers are reluctant to delegate, usually because of misapprehension, including:

- a belief that no one else can perform the delegated task as well as the manager;

- impatience with the delegation process (some managers believe that it is quicker to do the task themselves);
- fear that the delegatee will succeed at the delegated task, and the manager's position will then be threatened (if someone else can do the manager's work, why is the manager needed?);
- controlling behaviors that are not amenable to change, for example, managers who must oversee and be involved in every little task;
- fear that the delegatee will fail and that this failure will reflect badly upon the manager's own position within the organization;
- fear that the manager will be passed over for promotion in favor of delegatees who have performed delegated tasks well; and
- fear that managerial power and influence will be decreased if managerial tasks and responsibilities are delegated.

Sometimes managerial work accumulates until the manager does not have time to delegate; for example, in order to delegate, the manager must have time to explain the task to the delegatee. When time pressures have priority, managers tend not to delegate but to simply perform the tasks themselves. Sometimes well-intentioned managers recognize the pressures of time constraints and think that they will delegate appropriate tasks later when time is not such a problem. The problem with this logic is that later may never come. Delegation should be routine so the manager can readily delegate when work accu-mulates and time is tight. Ironically, delegation is most useful when the double pressures of accumulated work and time constraints merge. Managers who have not routinely delegated find that neither they nor their personnel feel comfortable with the process if it must be done under pressure.

Sometimes managers fail to delegate because they are ignorant of the benefits of delegating. Others fail at delegation because they fail to allot themselves sufficient time to explain the delegated task to delegatees. Further, some managerial judgment is required in delegating. A task cannot be appropriately delegated if it requires an employee to rapidly intervene in a situation and immediately make decisions. If a task is routine and time is not important, the task can be appropriately delegated.

Some managers do not provide delegatees with adequate information, do not delegate sufficient authority or do not provide adequate human and other organizational resources to accomplish the delegated tasks successfully. Some managers communicate the nature of the delegated task clearly, but many systematically undermine the process by interfering with the delegatee's performance or by inappropriately providing solutions that the delegatee could have deduced alone had the manager resisted the temptation to help. There is a genuine distinction between helping by providing answers and encouraging an employee to independently think through and creatively solve problems.

Some managers are unable to let their subordinates fail or partially succeed and thus learn from their mistakes. Some seem to be unaware of the need to groom subordinates so that the organization will always have an internal pool of human resources from which to select successive generations of leaders. Consider the following situation. A purchasing department employing twenty people was administered by a manager who was consistently unable to delegate. This manager handled all major accounts himself and closely monitored the processing of all other accounts. One day on his way to work the manager was involved in a serious automobile accident, which caused his absence for six weeks. During his absence, no one in his office was able to locate important accounts readily, respond to vendor queries, make timely decisions on important outstanding accounts or comprehend the highly individualized style of record keeping and notations that the manager used. The fact that no one in the purchasing department had been groomed to handle even part of the manager's responsibilities contributed to the chaos that the department experienced in his absence. Hospital administration until then had been unaware of the circumstances in the purchasing department. This crisis caused hospital administration to re-evaluate the oversight procedures for each department's operations and implement systems of organizational checks and balances to prevent the situation from recurring.

Employee attitudes resulting in problems with delegation

Some employees feel that they should receive additional compensation when they assume additional responsibilities. Some view extra responsibilities as an extra burden. Some employees are not sufficiently motivated or interested in expanding their horizons or enriching their jobs and are determined to function at the minimum acceptable level.

The escalating cost of health care and the health care industry's present cost-consciousness is resulting in reduced employee resistance to delegation. However, although employees may be more willing to perform delegated tasks, some delegatees still perform poorly. When this occurs, managers need to scrutinize each situation to determine where problems in the delegation process may have occurred. Phases of the delegation process are illustrated in Figure 2. Problems may arise at any phase of this process.

DECISION MAKING AND DELEGATION

Decisions must be made before tasks can be delegated. Some managers have difficulty making decisions for a variety of reasons: they are afraid of making the wrong decision; they fear repercussions if they make a poor decision; they are not risk takers; they lack adequate information on which to make an informed, timely decision; or their leadership

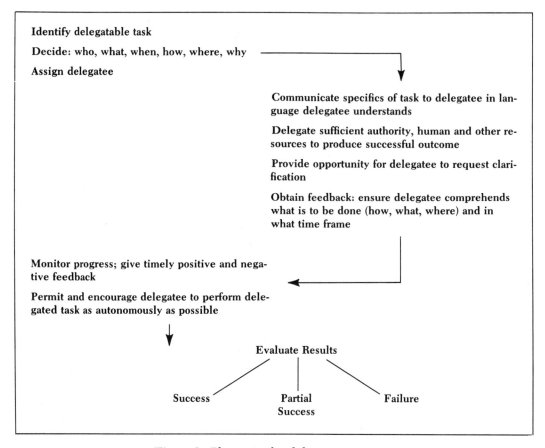

Figure 2. Phases in the delegation process.

style does not promote sound decision-making behavior patterns (for example, laissez-faire leaders typically have difficulty with this aspect of the managerial role).[6,7]

Sometimes an employee who occupies a managerial slot is simply not a "doer"—some employees are more appropriately suited to organizational positions where their primary responsibilities are to conceptualize, design potential organizational systems and carefully ponder the pros and cons of various alternative op-

tions. This is not to say that managers and administrators must not have these same abilities. However, managers must have the ability and the temperament to *institute* ideas and systems, monitor progress, intervene in problems when necessary, and continually seek ways to improve cost-efficient operations. In today's cost-cutting market, health care managers must demonstrate an orientation toward achieving goals. Managers who are unable to do this tend to experience sustained difficulty with both decision making and delegation and may have short-lived managerial careers.

Guidelines for effective decision making

When making a decision, a manager must assess the situation.
- Who will be directly and indirectly affected by this decision?
- What is the time frame for this decision?
- If this decision is implemented, what will be the likely responses?
- What alternative options or strategies are available?
- Is this decision best made with subordinate or staff input, or is it one that is primarily the prerogative of the manager?
- What are the risks involved with this decision? Are there any legal or other risk factors that should be considered? Will anyone be harmed by this decision?
- Is the decision likely to be accepted or rejected by those it will affect? If resistance is probable, how can it be lessened? Prevented? Responded to effectively?

Making decisions is a daily part of every manager's job. Few administrative decisions are of a life and death nature and few are perfect in execution or outcome. However, we live in a world of imperfects, where issues and situations are seldom clear cut. Managers must seek a tolerable comfort level in decision making and

learn to live with or accept the results of their decisions. Experienced managers realize that they will make bad decisions from time to time in spite of their best efforts. The seasoned manager will accept this as part of the management experience, will not permit it to undermine self-confidence, will try to learn from the experience and derive some benefit and personal growth from it and will continue to work toward goals.

Principles of effective delegation

Delegation is a learned art that is enhanced by repetition and adherence to some basic managerial strategies.
- Decide before delegating which tasks are routine and therefore appropriate for delegating and which cannot be delegated.
- Delegate tasks that have a high probability of being successfully accomplished.
- Delegate to the lowest employee level at which the task can be accomplished.
- Schedule sufficient time to communicate specifics of the task to the delegatee (e.g., who, what where, how, when, why), use language the delegatee can understand, ask for feedback on what is to be accomplished and provide the delegatee with the opportunity to ask questions.
- Delegate sufficient resources and authority to enable the delegatee to succeed.
- Support delegates but give them

the leeway to accomplish the task autonomously.

- Provide timely positive and negative feedback to delegatees during the delegation process, and monitor progress on a timely basis.
- Set up a routine, timely system of monitoring multifaceted or multiphased projects that have been delegated (e.g., designing a multidisciplinary patient health care plan or revised quality assurance system) or projects or tasks that have been delegated to a team. This is absolutely essential. Regularly scheduled monitoring helps both the manager and the team to gauge progress and provides the manager with opportunities to intervene early if problems evolve and to demonstrate supervisory interest in the project and the team.
- Assess the reason for failures when delegatees consistently fail. If managerial weaknesses caused the problem, correct the weaknesses and try again. If employee resistance to accepting delegated tasks caused failure, counsel the employee and continue to delegate.
- Follow the same process when delegatees are only partially successful. Evaluate what happened but do be certain to commend the delegatee for the part that was successful.
- Provide regular follow-up and supervisory guidance throughout the entire delegation process;

this is crucial to ensuring delegatee successes.

Managers who fail to regularly monitor delegatees' progress toward achieving goals tend to provoke problems that would most likely have been preventable had timely managerial oversight occurred. Regular monitoring and follow-up with delegatees, providing both positive and negative feedback and establishing ground rules are important. Delegatees must know that the manager has certain expectations; however, they also must know that should difficulties in accomplishing goals arise, the manager is accessible and willing to provide appropriate supervisory support. These straightforward managerial strategies will determine the atmosphere in which delegation occurs as well as its outcomes.

Regular monitoring and follow-up with delegatees, providing both positive and negative feedback and establishing ground rules are important.

In addition to these guidelines, managers must be generous in recognizing delegatees who have performed delegated tasks exceptionally well. For example, a small local hospital asked one of its employees to put together an in-house marketing campaign for the annual United Way kickoff activities. The employee did an outstanding job on this delegated task, designing colorful posters and placing them in highly visible locations throughout the hospital, ordering United Way kickoff buttons and pins, preparing news briefs for the hospital's newsletter and forming United Way teams composed of staff-level employees for every major hospital unit and department. With enthusiasm and commitment this employee single-handedly organized one of the most successful United Way contribution years in the hospital's history. One might ask what recognition was accorded this unusual employee. Hospital administration acknowledged this person in several ways: A special letter of commendation was written by the president and placed in her personnel file, a special acknowledgement accompanied by the employee's photograph was included in the hospital's newsletter, the hospital honored the employee at a special brunch and presented her with a gift certificate for dinner for two at one of the prestigious local restaurants and with a plaque citing her contributions to the hospital's United Way effort.

Consider another case history, one with a far less positive outcome. Administrators of a 325-bed hospital decided to improve the hospital's quality assurance program by increasing staff involvement. The hospital was operating under the prospective payment system, was competing with several other local hospitals within the same 50-mile radius, had sustained a decrease in occupancy rates over the previous 12 months and had an average institutional image in the community. Some of the problems confronting hospital administrators were: longer patient stays than were allowable under the diagnostic related group major diagnostic categories; demoralized clinical personnel whose diminished levels of self-esteem were reflected in their appearance, attitude and the abrupt manner in which many of them related to patients and patients' significant others; and denial of third party reimbursements or lower rates of reimbursement caused by documentation deficiencies or errors. The administration decided to change the membership of the institution's hospital-wide quality assurance committee to reflect more staff-level representatives while simultaneously decreasing representation from clinical department chiefs.

Volunteers to staff the quality assurance committee were aggressively recruited. Hospital administration emphasized that committee members would have the opportunity to make a positive difference not only in the quality of patient care but in the long-term viability of the institution and in working conditions for themselves and their fellow employees. The committee was reconstituted within a short time. New committee members brought different concerns and new perspectives to the quality of care issues being discussed, and more important, being staff-level employees who were directly involved in providing clinical services to patients, they provided a wide range of suggestions and insights about maximizing patient care services in a cost-efficient manner. The committee attacked its mission with enthusiasm and commitment. Members reviewed incident reports critically, reviewed multidisciplinary medical record documentation, studied patient outcomes and experiences during hospitalization, designed brief surveys to assess patient, visitor and staff satisfaction and followed up with all known patient, visitor and staff complaints.

Some of the recommendations and proposals provided by the staff-level committee members not only proved to be effective in assuring quality but also resulted in cost savings to the hospital—an unexpected benefit. Six months after the committee began operating, hospital administration noted that the number and types of both major and minor patient complaints had decreased and savings because of: decreased length of patient stay, improved documentation leading to maximal reimbursement by third party payers, improved levels of patient satisfaction, decreased staff dissatisfaction and a slight increase in bed occupancy rates, were considerable. Further, steadily rising annual turnover rates for personnel (particularly nursing personnel) that had been consistently in the 30 percent to 35 percent range had begun to decrease. These remarkable changes had occurred in a relatively short time and it seemed that the work and persistence of the new committee were producing astounding results, largely because of staff-level members' input and efforts. One would surmise that hospital administration would vigorously acknowledge the excellent results produced by this committee. However, hospital administration assumed a wait-and-see posture and informed the committee that, while the perceived changes were very fine, it doubted whether the committee could sustain its level of productivity and suspected that the improvements may have been just a fluke. As could be predicted, the committee is entering its second six months with a demoralized spirit and the committee's further efforts are unlikely to produce continued outstanding results. From an organizational perspective, the governing board would be prudent to reconstitute the top-level hospital administration, as the problem in this instance lies neither with inappropriate delegation nor unsuccessful delegation, but with the unenlightened responses from top administrators when delegatees produce superlative results.

•   •   •

Successful delegation cannot be brought about by discussion contained on a few printed pages. Successful delegation can only be achieved by managers who decide to delegate, live with the results, assess and improve their delegating skills and continue to delegate as a matter of developing and strengthening their approach to informed, progressive management of human resources in health care systems.

REFERENCES

1. Caruth, D., and Middlebrook, B. "How to Delegate Successfully." *Supervisory Management* 28 (February 1983): 36–42.

2. Volante, E. "Mastering the Managerial Art of Delegation." *Journal of Nursing Administration* 4, no. 1 (1974): 20–22.

3. Ford, R. "Delegation Without Fear." *Supervisory Management* 28 (July 1983): 2–8.

4. Kobert, N. *Aggressive Management Style.* Englewood Cliffs, N.J.: Prentice-Hall, 1981, pp. 155–176.

5. Winslow, E. "Step Aside and Let a Pro Do It!" *Supervisory Management* 27, no. 6 (1982): 2–5.

6. Bailey, J., Faan, E., and Hendricks, D. "Decisions, Decisions: Guidelines for Making Them More Easily." *Nursing Life* 2, no. 4 (1982): 45–47.

7. Delaney, W. "Why Are People Indecisive?" *Supervisory Management* 27, no. 12 (1982): 26–30.

The supervisor's role in the disciplinary and grievance procedure

Norman Metzger
Vice-President for Labor Relations
The Mount Sinai Medical Center
New York, New York

RARELY DOES A week or even a day go by in which the supervisor is not called on to consider disciplining an employee in the department. The rationalization for the supervisor's role in the disciplinary process is that it comes with the turf. The supervisor must take corrective action when an employee is chronically late, has an absenteeism problem, disregards a rule or policy of the institution, refuses to follow an order, is unproductive, is uncooperative or in some other way does not meet the standards of the institution.

In reviewing the long list of breaches of institutional policy and negative employee actions, it is clear that the supervisor has a continuing responsibility to take corrective action. More often than not, the act of disciplining is conceived of as punishment, but meting out punishment may be far less difficult than sustain-

Health Care Superv, 1983,2(1),77–86
© 1983 Aspen Publishers, Inc.

ing the action that may have been taken in the grievance procedure.

It is in the application of that procedure that a supervisor will have to prove that he or she had "good and just cause" for disciplining an employee. A penalty imposed by the supervisor will not be modified by an arbitrator unless it is shown to have been clearly arbitrary, capricious, discriminatory or excessive relative to the events in the case. The key point to understand about the limitation on the supervisor's right to discipline is that administration may discipline up through discharge *only* for sufficient and appropriate reasons.

CORRECTIVE DISCIPLINE

Before considering the supervisor's role in the grievance procedure, consider the pertinence of the adage, "forearmed is forewarned." To sustain the action in the arbitration process, it is well to be aware of Justin's Rules of Corrective Discipline:[1]

1. To be meaningful discipline must be corrective, not punitive.
2. When you discipline one, you discipline all.
3. Corrective discipline satisfies the rule of equality of treatment by enforcing equally among all employees' established rules, safety practices and responsibility on the job.
4. It is the job of the supervisor, not the shop steward, to make the worker tow the line or increase efficiency.
5. Just cause or any comparable

standard for justifying disciplinary action under the labor contract consists of three parts:

- Did the employee breach the rule or commit the offense charged against him or her?
- Did the employee's act or misconduct warrant corrective action or punishment?
- Is the penalty just and appropriate to the act or offense as corrective punishment?

6. The burden of proof rests on the supervisor. He or she must justify each of the three parts that make up the standard or just cause under the labor contract.

Most arbitrators who are called on to adjudicate grievances have set up criteria for the sustaining of discharges (the most common management action submitted to third party binding arbitration). For supervisors, these criteria are as follows:

1. You must prove that the act you have alleged the employee participated in actually occurred and that it warranted discharge.
2. You must prove beyond a reasonable doubt that such actions were not condoned in the past, that you have consistently disciplined employees for similar actions, that the employee was specifically warned of the consequences of his or her actions and that progressive disciplining, including written warnings and suspensions, preceded the action if it was not severe enough to be punished by discharge at the first occurrence.

3. If warnings were present, you must prove that the employee made no genuine effort to heed such warnings, even though you informed him or her of the consequences of continued misconduct.

4. As Justin pointed out, you must demonstrate that the employee was not singled out for disparate treatment, and that the rule of equality of treatment was respected.[2]

5. When dealing with a long-service employee, the case must be stronger. You must demonstrate that the action was not transitory but was part of a consistent and recurrent pattern that is unlikely to change.

Positive discipline encompasses the following sound supervisory practices:

1. Inform *all* employees of the rules and the penalties. The "why" of the rule is just as important as the "what."

2. Do not play the game of "Do as I say, not as I do." Set a good example. Employees look to their supervisors for fairness in application of the rules.

3. Do not jump before you look. Get all of the facts. Keep uppermost in your mind the adage that there are at least two sides to every story.

4. Beware of incomplete facts or misleading appearances. Judge an act within its context. Look for the least obvious motives and reasons.

5. Move quickly but not hastily. Do not let selected instances of misbehavior develop into habits.

6. Corrective discipline should be meted out in private.

7. Objectivity, fairness and consistency are the hallmarks of positive, corrective disciplinary action.

8. Throughout the disciplinary process, remain aware of the goal of the process: to correct improper behavior and to salvage the employee.

9. Use punishment only as the last resort.

THE GRIEVANCE PROCEDURE

What is the grievance procedure and what is it intended to do? Arbitrator Herbert Marx would answer this question as follows:

The significance of the grievance procedure leading up to the arbitration hearing, is often grossly underestimated. The major purpose of the grievance procedure is to resolve disputes bilaterally before they get to arbitration. Too often this principle is forgotten or disregarded and the parties use the grievance procedure simply as a means either to expedite the dispute to arbitration or to get the one party to concede because it does not wish to undergo the risk, inconvenience and expense of arbitration.[3]

Understanding the purpose

Unfortunately, the grievance procedure is often misused. Marx directs attention to the real purpose of that mechanism—to resolve disputes bilaterally. A supervisor assumes a heavy burden when assuming the role of adjudicator of grievances. The major part of the burden is to facilitate the identification of employee complaints in order to settle them peacefully. Festering dissatisfaction is far more dangerous than the number of grievances that inappropriately come to the surface for political or destructive purposes. In the final analysis, a supervisor does not lose by encouraging the processing of grievances.

It has been proven time and time again that the huge majority of grievances are settled at the first step, between the employee and his or her representative and the first-line supervisor. The reason for this is quite clear. Many grievances are not bona fide when weighed against the legal definition in a labor contract or in a personnel policy manual. Rather, they are often a search for an answer, a direction or a sympathetic ear.

The grievance procedure is an integral part of the management communication network. It must not be so cumbersome that it discourages submissions rather than encouraging them. It is a useful, necessary and productive management tool *if* it involves fact finding, objective evaluation and equitable decision making.

The grievance procedure is as valid in nonunion settings as it is where it is mandated in a labor contract. In a nonunionized health care institution, the supervisor often is the day-to-day interpreter of personnel policy and the dispenser of discipline. Although the collective bargaining agreement enshrines due process, the concept of due process is not limited solely to unionized relationships. Due process should be equally encouraged in nonunion settings. A grievance procedure is useful for all employees. To defend the lack of grievance machinery on the basis of a misguided belief that no grievances exist is unrealistic. Grievance machinery or not, employees will have problems.

Another fallacy is that an informal procedure fondly referred to as the *open-door policy* can be substituted for a formal grievance process. Can an employee at a lower level truly express his or her frustrations, fears or needs to a person in a much higher position who appears to be isolated from the very problem of the work place? Is it not true that many executives find such activities to be an imposition on their busy schedules? It is only with a published formal grievance procedure that problems come to the surface and are adjudicated fairly, expeditiously and, in the main, with productivity uninterrupted.

The typical grievance procedure contains four steps, three within the institution and the final step an appeal outside the institution. The first-line supervisor is the management representative at step one of the grievance procedure and is usually, in a unionized environment, faced with the employee and his or her representative. Step two provides for the appeal of the first-line supervisor's decision to a department head or a member of management in an echelon above the first-line supervisor. Step three finds a union official representing the employee. Management is usually represented at this step by a labor relations representative. Step four is the final appeal, to an arbitrator.

It is critical that step one include a meeting between the employee and the first-line supervisor. In the final analysis, it is some action of the first-line supervisor that the employee is referring to in submitting a formal grievance. It is a clear duty of the

---

In the final analysis, it is some action of the supervisor that the employee is referring to in submitting a formal grievance.

---

institution to adjust grievances promptly and, preferably, at the first step in the procedure. Indeed, it is not unlikely, with sensitive supervisors, that the overwhelming majority of grievances can and should be informally adjusted and disposed of at the first-line supervisor's level.

The supervisor has three major responsibilities in the grievance procedure. The first is to hear grievances. The second is to investigate the facts. The third is to evaluate and decide, finally communicating the decision to the employee.

Hearing the grievance

In hearing the grievance, it is strongly suggested that a clinical ap-proach be taken. This approach attempts to get to the heart of the problem. It includes the extensive search for the fundamental determinant of the grievance, rather than the acceptance, at face value, of its surface rationale. There is a need for an empathetic probe into the circumstances and causes of the grievance. Many gripes submitted to the grievance procedure are not bona fide grievances because they concern situations that are not specifically covered by a collective bargaining agreement or by a personnel policy manual.

When hearing a grievance, it is essential to practice good listening habits. These include providing an uninterrupted platform for the employee or his or her representative to present the grievance, not prejudging at this stage of the process, providing for a cooling off period if the situation is emotion-laden, and protecting the dignity of all parties to the process.

After the employee has presented his or her side of the case (or the employee's representative has done so), ask questions until you completely understand the specifics of the grievance and the true agenda. It is essential that you not be predisposed or argumentative, if at all possible, in response to the employee's answers. The hearing room may be a heated one, but you must stay calm.

Very often complaints reflect dissatisfaction in areas other than those under discussion, so attempting to establish the hidden agenda is critical. It is essential to find out what is really bothering the employee. It may be necessary to ask for further explanation or discussion.

Nothing should be promised at this time other than a careful investigation. Keep to the time schedule in answering the grievance. The supervisor should not mislead the employee by promising to do something about the complaint unless remedial action is truly called for. There may be occasions when a quick response is indicated on the basis of an absolute certainty as to the facts, but in most instances a hasty decision can be disastrous.

Investigating the facts

As stated, very few grievances can be adjudicated on the spot. An interest in prompt handling of grievances should not compromise this investigatory stage. It is during this stage that emotional arguments must be filtered out and set aside and a study of the facts undertaken. You may have to interview other employees who were involved in the issue at hand. You should review relevant records. You may have to study the grievance in a general way to ascertain whether it is related to other grievances that recently have been filed.

You should also investigate the employee's motivations. It is essential to determine whether you are dealing with a habitual complainer. The records become important; documentation is at the foundation of appropriate grievance administration. What do the records show about previous disciplinary action, if any, and about

attendance, punctuality, job performance and other behavior and characteristics? It is during this stage that the supervisor steps back from the problem to gain objectivity. Beware of establishing precedents or creating new policy. You should review the clauses of the contract or of the personnel policy manual so that you understand the perimeters of your decision-making ability.

It cannot be repeated too often that you should look for information concerning previous settlements of similar grievances and relevant policy or contract interpretation. Checking with another supervisor, the personnel manager or a labor relations manager is not a sign of weakness. On the contrary, precedence becomes extremely important. A hasty decision may provide a precedent with far-reaching impact. Many a supervisor has found that a hasty or careless decision about a relatively minor occurrence becomes important later in a situation having more serious consequences.

During this investigatory stage, additional considerations should be sought. Is there anything that might be affecting the employee's on-the-job behavior? Is there a less obvious reason for the employee's discontent? Often the surface cause of the grievance may differ markedly from underlying causes. If you can discover the underlying causes of grievances, rather than reacting to external appearances, you can start solving real labor relations problems.

Making a decision

Grievance handling can be looked at from two vantage points, the legalistic and the clinical. The legalistic approach emphasizes form and mechanics. It focuses on accepting or dismissing grievances on the basis of whether they are within the contract.

The clinical approach attempts to get to the heart of the problem. It involves an empathetic probe into the actual circumstances and causes of the grievance. It includes an intensive search for the fundamental determinants of a grievance, rather than acceptance, at face value, of the surface rationale. It need not be the only approach; the clinical approach can augment the legalistic approach. The two approaches are not mutually exclusive.

To review, management's responsibility for the grievance procedure entails three primary functions:

1. investigating the material facts of grievances;
2. discussing and answering grievances; and
3. analyzing grievances to determine their basic causes.

To discharge grievance-handling responsibilities properly, you must be constantly aware that your first task is to investigate, not evaluate. The time for evaluation comes after the facts have been investigated.

When you are ready to evaluate, it is often helpful to discuss and test your solutions to the problem with others. Checking out your hunch, your conclusion or your options with others who are in a position to assess their probable impact is a wise idea. Ask another supervisor, ask your department head and consult with the personnel executive. Ask how this type of problem has been handled in the past. Consultation is a sign of caution, not of indecision. You will not be criticized for reviewing your options with others if you have assembled the facts carefully and have approached the grievance objectively.

At this point, the decision should be made and put into written form. If you have done your job properly, you have studied the grievance in a general way, have analyzed the specific parts of the grievance, have studied the employee involved, and have looked carefully for additional considerations. It is well to remember that a sympathetic no often goes a much longer way than a harsh yes.

If you have carefully investigated the facts and unemotionally analyzed your findings, there is no reason to be concerned about the appropriateness of your decision. However, it is essential that you detail the reasons why you have come to your conclusion. Limit your comments to the specific complaint. Ensure that the answer deals with the specific grievance at hand. If a grievance has merit and an error has been made, admit this to the employee and indicate your intention to take immediate corrective action.

If the employee's grievance has no merit and you must deny the charges or turn down the request, attempt to obtain the employee's understanding of how you came to your decision and his or her acceptance of that decision. Remember, *you* have made the decision. It is not appropriate to pass the buck by placing the blame on your department head. You can gain the respect of employees even while denying their grievances. During the communication of your decision, your attention should be directed to that area of responsibility—explaining why and obtaining understanding.

PITFALLS OF GRIEVANCE HANDLING

To review the mistakes of others is to be forewarned and forearmed. There are many dangers to be encountered in fulfilling your responsibility as a critical participant in the grievance procedure. Over the years, the author has uncovered the following key pitfalls:

1. The supervisor has an inadequate understanding of the union agreement. It is your responsibility to review the contract and the personnel policy manual before making a decision. You can be certain that your union counterpart (the delegate) knows the employee's right and knows the contract from cover to cover. Do not commit a procedural or technical error because you did not know what the contract contained or because you were unsure of the meaning of a specific clause. Check with an authority if you experience any doubt.

2. The investigation is slipshod, hasty, subjective and likely to foster a self-fulfilling prophesy. It is essential that you not rely on hearsay or judge the book by its cover. Do not be impulsive and do not hurry. Also, be aware of contractual time limits that may govern your responsibility in answering the grievance.

3. A supervisor may misinterpret the facts. Do not be confused by the facts, but rather be aware of their meaning. There is no room for emotional interpretations of what occurred.

4. Supervisors are often not aware of a change in conditions. Circumstances do change, and therefore you should not automatically continue to do things today in the same way that you did them yesterday. You must adjust to change, and you must consider the grievance carefully on the basis of new conditions. It is equally important to recognize that there must occasionally be exceptions to the rules. If the imposition of a rule in a particular set of circumstances would be absolutely unfair to an employee, you should consider making an exception.

5. The supervisor fails to act promptly. Although haste is to be avoided, if an employee believes you are giving him or her the runaround, resentment will

grow. Supervisors who get the reputation of "holding the ball" on grievances instead of keeping it rolling will win no employee loyalty. Grievances

---

Supervisors who get the reputation of "holding the ball" on grievances instead of keeping it rolling will win no employee loyalty.

---

should be adjusted promptly, preferably at the first step.

6. Supervisors who fail to look ahead often stumble. Try to anticipate problems that might upset employees, for example, changes in the content of the job or the introduction of a new method or a new piece of equipment. In anticipating such problems, you will prepare yourself and prepare the employee. A prepared employee is more receptive and less likely to have a complaint.

GUIDELINES FOR EFFECTIVE GRIEVANCE HANDLING

The supervisor is the key to the effective handling of grievances. Most grievances are settled at the first step by the first-line supervisor. Here are some tips to assist you in administering the grievance procedure:

1. Workers are people, and people have individual needs. Keep in mind, when you are dealing with people's problems, that each person is unique.

2. At the heart of a sound supervisor–employee relationship is a firm commitment on the part of the supervisor to maintain and preserve the dignity of employees. This may be difficult in the emotion-charged environment of the grievance procedure, but it is essential that you treat all employees fairly and consider their dignity in all dealings even when adverse relations exist.

3. Try to anticipate problems and actions that may cause irritation and therefore result in grievances. By anticipating problems, you will minimize them.

4. Many grievances occur because of inadequate employee training. Employees who are inept are often unhappy. Those who know that they are doing well are less likely to be frustrated. This is of particular relevance in dealing with new employees.

5. Make certain that your orders or instructions are clear and that you include the "why" as well as the "how."

6. Progressive disciplining is at the heart of reducing grievances. It is corrective in nature and based on an objective, equitable and consistent application. The majority of grievances stem from real or perceived inequality of treatment.

7. If an employee has a grievance, it does not matter whether the

problem is covered in the personnel policy manual or the labor contract. It is real to the employee, and you must deal with it. Do not belittle employees, and never underestimate them. The supervisor's role in taking disciplinary action and applying the grievance procedure can be difficult and time consuming. However, few other supervisory activities are ever more important in the ongoing task of maintaining a smoothly functioning department.

REFERENCES

1. Justin, J.J. *How to Manage with a Union, Book 1.* New York: Industrial Relations Workshop Seminars, 1969, pp. 294–95, 301–02.

2. Ibid.

3. Marx, H.L. Jr. "Arbitration from the Arbitrator's View." In *HANDBOOK of Health Care Human Resources Management* edited by N. Metzger. Rockville, Md. Aspen Systems Corporation, 1981, p. 830.

Team-building techniques for the health care supervisor

Jerry L. Norville
Professor/Associate Chairman
Department of Health
Administration
Medical College of Virginia
Virginia Commonwealth
University
Richmond, Virginia

IMPROVING EMPLOYEE productivity while maintaining service level and quality in the wake of recent changes in reimbursement for patient care is the single greatest challenge facing health care supervisors today. Meeting this challenge requires innovative leadership, high levels of employee commitment and a high degree of mutual support among members of the health care team. The nation's health care supervisors can and will meet this challenge with the same commitment and vigor they have applied to similar challenges, but they will need the full support of their work groups.

THE SUPERVISOR'S CHALLENGE

Major advances in technology, a proliferation of specialization and a marked shift in the locus of delivery

Health Care Superv, 1983,2(1),37–52
© 1983 Aspen Publishers, Inc.

of medical care to more formal organizational settings have resulted in greater levels of interdependence for physicians and the many professionals who support them.[1] In essence, work in health care has become more structured. It is now more intensely specialized and grouped by functions, departments and work units.

As the work related to the delivery of health care services has become more differentiated, problems of effectively integrating the performance of many diverse occupations and professional groups have become a major concern of those responsible for supervising health care personnel. Productivity levels in many health care organizations have not reached their potential and have not met management expectations.

Because there is a limit in a labor-intensive environment to the gains in productivity that can be made through advanced technology, health care supervisors must grapple with ways to improve productivity and ensure quality care. Given this situation, the thrust of today's efforts to improve productivity must be directed toward improving the performance of work groups. The emphasis of such efforts must be at the level of the first-line supervisor.

MULTIPLE BENEFITS OF TEAM BUILDING

Given the interdependencies and complexities of the health care personnel force and health care organizations, one effective approach to achieving improvements in productivity as well as in quality is to apply team-building processes in the health care setting. Team building, or team development, is a systematic, planned group process aimed at unifying a group of employees with common objectives into an effective and efficiently functioning work unit.[2] The process is designed to assist the work group in becoming more adept at pursuing its objectives and in identifying as well as resolving its own work-related problems. Team building is a proven, effective technique for achieving high levels of work group performance.

The amalgamation of individual talents to achieve an orchestrated effort in planning and achieving departmental objectives is the first-line supervisor's purpose in developing an effective health care team. In essence, the team is built so that the level of cooperative action by each team member contributes to a total effect greater than the sum of individual contributions. This is referred to as the synergistic effect.

Faced with the challenge of doing more with less, health care supervisors can realize two major benefits through the application of a systematic team-building process. Team building can lead to higher levels of productivity while meeting expected levels of quality. Team building can improve the work climate, enhance supervisor–employee relationships and increase employee satisfaction.

Team building can yield a number

of additional benefits. For example, a well-developed work team will perform complex tasks more effectively. It will also be more responsive to change as well as to unforeseen contingencies. Moreover, it will exhibit a collective strength that enhances its support of the organization. Finally, a well-developed team will be less likely to demonstrate such counterproductive behavior as absenteeism or tardiness, or to be involved in incidents requiring disciplinary action.

TEAM BUILDING AS A LONG-TERM STRATEGY

Those people who read the title of this article and hope to find a panacea for the many human problems of supervision will be disappointed. There simply is no panacea. Those people who read this article expecting to find a list of quick-fix prescriptions for the day-to-day problems of employee productivity, quality and satisfaction will also be disappointed. There simply are no such fast cures. However, those people who are realistic and who have a strong commitment to seeking new ways of improving as health care supervisors, thus improving the work group for which they are responsible, will want to apply team-building techniques.

Building an effective team-oriented work group is neither a simple nor a quick process. The process of information gathering, group assessment, plan development, implementation and evaluation of the results requires a great deal of a supervisor's

time and effort, but the personal rewards and the organizational benefits to be derived from developing an effective work group are many. In the opinion of those who have done it successfully, the results are more than adequate compensation for the time and effort required in applying team-building concepts.

TEAM BUILDING IN PERSPECTIVE

Before initiating any process focused on developing people, it is important to understand how it relates to other group processes. In their quest for answers to the problems of productivity, quality and employee satisfaction, behavioral scientists have recommended a plethora of approaches. Some of these recommended techniques for improving motivation and employee satisfaction focus on modifying behavior in the entire organization, whereas others are aimed at small work groups or individual employees.

Examples of techniques that have been applied at the work group level include:

- job enrichment or job enlargement approaches in which jobs are redesigned to increase the levels of task variety;
- semi-autonomous work group approaches in which employees are given considerable freedom in deciding who will accomplish particular tasks;
- survey feedback meetings where employees discuss the results of

surveys relating to their work and attitudes;

- transactional analysis sessions focused on the analysis and improvement of the communication process;
- quality circles in which groups of employees meet voluntarily to discuss, analyze and develop solutions to production and quality problems; and
- team-building processes that focus on simultaneous development of the group's effectiveness and on improving the work tasks of the group.

These techniques assume that the majority of employees have a desire to apply more of their abilities to their work, and that when they are not permitted to apply their talents work becomes less satisfying. It also assumes that failure to tap the potential of its employees makes the organization less effective than it could otherwise be. Given these assumptions, all of these approaches advocate that supervisors share their power with employees, that employees be given greater autonomy and that employees be encouraged to participate more fully in the affairs of the work group. Team building includes these same assumptions and advocates the same shared power and increased level of employee participation.

WORK GROUPS IN PERSPECTIVE

Having put the team development concept in its proper perspective, at-

tention can now be focused on putting the work group in perspective. Before initiating a team development process with subordinates, the health care supervisor should first possess a fundamental knowledge of work group behavior and an understanding of his or her role as the appointed leader of the work group. To strengthen such understanding, some important concepts of both work groups and individual supervisory behavior must be reviewed.

The nature of a work group is largely determined by such factors as the size of the group, longevity of the members, formal and informal reward or recognition systems, general group expectations of the leader and of each other, role behavior of formal and informal group leaders and extent of balance in downward, upward and lateral communications and personal interaction.[3] Employees bring to the work group unique backgrounds that include past experiences and education as well as present knowledge, skills and attitudes. In performing their tasks, they must engage in certain required interactions with others in the immediate work group and often outside the immediate group. Job descriptions, policies and procedures largely dictate their required actions and interactions in this formal work group.

Formal and informal structures

It is necessary but not sufficient for a supervisor to understand only the formal structure and tasks of his or her area of responsibility. Supervisors must also fully understand and take into account the emergence of an informal structure within the work group that has its own unique set of social relationships. For example, new employees soon learn that, in addition to their formal job expectations as communicated through their job descriptions and through their supervisors, there exist separate work-group-developed expectations or norms regarding what constitutes acceptable group behavior both socially and in relation to the work itself.

Individuals tend to behave differently in groups than they do as individuals, because of the influence of group values. There is a strong pull from the group that generally results in individuals' conformance to group norms regarding work and social behavior. This informal social structure that emerges from the formal group structure serves important functions, including satisfaction of affiliation, security and self-esteem needs and as a means of establishing a frame of reference for behavior and interaction.

One key to effective group performance is achieving an appropriate balance between the formal and informal aspects of the group. If the informal leadership and social network are working against the supervisor, efficiency and effectiveness are likely

---

If the informal leadership and social network are working against the supervisor, efficiency and effectiveness are likely to be low.

---

to be low. If the supervisor is able to gain the support of the informal group and its leaders, then the work group is likely to demonstrate high levels of productivity and quality while also expressing job satisfaction.

Individual needs

Basically, there are two types of human relationships that are important in accounting for the productivity of work groups. First are those relationships that are influenced by actual similarities and differences in various backgrounds and personality traits of team members. Second are those relationships that are influenced by team members' perceptions of each other.[4]

Among the employees in the work group, as in all aspects of life, a full spectrum of attitudes and accompanying behaviors exists. Some employees are dedicated, ambitious, concerned with quality and productivity and generally supportive of the work group's mission. Others may be diffident, hostile, sullen, uncooperative or just plain lazy. Some employees will dislike their work; others would rather work than play. There is simply no single work style indicative of those who demonstrate peak performance versus those who do not perform well. We do know, however, that subverting some individual needs to those of the group is absolutely essential to a satisfying and productive work environment.[5]

An additional consideration in putting the work group in proper perspective is the behavior of the group's formal leader. The health care supervisor is the appointed leader of the work group. For the group leader, self-understanding is just as important as understanding the group. Supervisors bring to the work place certain assumptions about themselves as well as about their subordinates, certain attitudes about the job, certain self-interests to be satisfied and certain patterns of leadership or management style. These unique attributes may greatly influence the supervisor's performance.

Before considering team building for one's work group, it is essential to:

1. make positive assumptions about the value of human resources;
2. sincerely believe that the employees desire to assume greater levels of responsibility for themselves and their work;
3. be willing to share power with subordinates and encourage their genuine participation in decisions that affect them; and,
4. be willing to subordinate short-run self-interests to achieve the long-run benefits of team building.

If these positive aspects of team building are accepted and practiced, then it will more likely be possible to develop the level of teamwork desired of the particular work group.

BEHAVIORAL STAGES IN TEAM BUILDING

It is important to distinguish the steps in the team-building process from likely behavioral stages related to the process. Walton and Smith have identified the following five behavioral stages, which provide insight regarding possible behavior that might be manifested during team building.[6]

1. *Formation:* Commitment is tentative, and communications are guarded.
2. *Disequilibrium:* Ideals may conflict, and protectiveness may emerge.
3. *Role definition:* Team identity emerges, roles are clarified and communication becomes more open.
4. *Maturity:* High levels of cooperation, mutual support, productivity and satisfaction are evident.
5. *Maintenance:* Infusion of new ideas and challenges maintains team effectiveness.

These expected stages of behavior are normal aspects of team-building behavior and should be regarded as such.

Once an effective team is formed, maintenance becomes an important consideration. In the absence of new ideas and challenges, the work group may become complacent and less effective. According to Herzberg, pressures toward group identity, group thinking and group motivation may run counter to the belief that productivity depends on individual motivations. He believes that group solidarity can be a force, but it cannot sustain productivity. Although they must focus on team building, supervisors "cannot afford to assume that individual competence and commitment are dispensable."[7] It is therefore highly important that individual identity and motivation be maintained as the core of an effective work team. The team maintenance phase is thus an ongoing effort.

WORK PROCESS STEPS IN TEAM BUILDING

In all human interactions, there are two major dimensions, content and process. Content refers to the subject matter or tasks of the work group. Process refers to the dynamics of what is happening to and between work group members. The team-building approach presented in Figure 1 focuses on the behavioral processes of the work group and on the work content of the group's efforts. An effective team-building effort will improve both the work interrelationships and the actual work output of the group.

Identify and compare characteristics

Assuming that the work group is already defined, the first step in developing the teamwork process is to identify model characteristics of an effective work group. Francis and Young define an effective work team as one that produces outstanding results, succeeds in achieving despite difficulties, has members that "feel responsible for the output of their team" and has members that "act to clear difficulties standing in their way."[8] Effective task perfor-

mance, a clearly defined contribution to the organization and high morale are some of the hallmarks of a "team" as opposed to a traditional work group.

Many factors influence the performance of a work group. Shonk has provided a useful list of factors.[9] These include: (1) the extent of successful interactions with other elements of the organization, (2) the goals of the group and how well these are understood and supported, (3) the individual roles of group members and how well these have been clarified, (4) the specific work processes that dictate interactions and interdependencies among group members and (5) the quality of human relationships between individuals within the group. If all these factors are positive, the result is likely to be an effective teamwork-oriented work group.

Francis and Young have developed one of the most comprehensive descriptions of an effective team.[10] A summary of their model is presented (see box) so that health care supervisors can consider their own work groups in relation to these essential elements of an effective work team.

As the next step in the process, the 12 model characteristics should be compared with the actual characteristics of a work group. It is recommended that initially the supervisors do this personally and then perform a group comparison with members of the work group. The purpose of this comparison is to reveal the strengths of the group as well as areas needing attention.

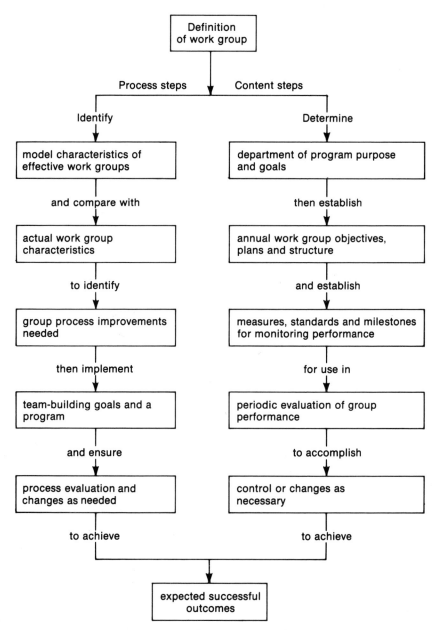

Figure 1. Sequential steps in team building.

Identify and develop goals

As a result of the comparison of the model with actual performance per-ceptions of the work group, the supervisor and team members should jointly identify group process improvements needed and establish

Characteristics of Effective Work Teams

Appropriate leadership. The team manager has the skills and intention to develop a team approach and allocates time to team-building activities. Management in the team is seen as a shared function. Individuals other than the manager are given the opportunity to exercise leadership when their skills are appropriate to the needs of the team.

Suitable membership. Team members are individually qualified and capable of contributing the "mix" of skills and characteristics that provide an appropriate balance.

Commitment to the team. Team members feel a sense of individual commitment to the aims and purposes of the team. They are willing to devote personal energy to building the team and supporting other team members. When working outside the team boundaries, the members feel a sense of belonging to and representing the team.

Constructive climate. The team has developed a climate in which people feel relaxed, able to be direct and open, and prepared to take risks.

Concern to achieve. The team is clear about its objectives, which are felt to be worthwhile. It sets targets of performance that are felt to be stretching but achievable. Energy is mainly devoted to the achievement of results, and team performance is reviewed frequently to see where improvements can be made.

Clear corporate role. The team has contributed to corporate planning and has a distinct and productive role within the overall organization.

Effective work methods. The team has developed lively, systematic, and effective ways to solve problems together.

Well-organized team procedures. Roles are clearly defined, communication patterns are well developed, and administrative procedures support a team approach.

Critique without rancor. Team and individual errors and weaknesses are examined, without personal attack, to enable the group to learn from its experience.

Well-developed individuals. Team members are deliberately developed and the team can cope with strong individual contributions.

Creative strength. The team has the capacity to create new ideas through the interactions of its members. Some innovative risk taking is rewarded, and the team will support new ideas from individual members or from outside. Good ideas are followed through into action.

Positive intergroup relations. Relationships with other teams have been systematically developed to provide open personal contact and identify where joint working may give maximum pay off. There is regular contact and review of joint or collective priorities with other teams. Individuals are encouraged to contact and work with members of other teams.

Reprinted with permission from D. Francis and D. Young, *Improving Work Groups: A Practical Manual for Team Building,* San Diego, CA: Pfeiffer & Company, 1979. Used with permission.

tentative teamwork improvement goals. These goals should be considered tentative until they are fully supported by the group through consensus-building sessions. It is essential that employees in the group voluntarily set these goals and commit themselves to a team-building program.

Employees who feel that their

opinions matter, whose suggestions are acknowledged and whose efforts and overall contribution to the work group are recognized feel good about themselves. In turn, they will probably care more about their jobs, their fellow employees, the institution in which they work and its patients.

Planning the team-building program requires a great deal of detailed effort. To assist in initially planning the effort, a flow chart has been included as Figure 2. The questions asked in Figure 2 and the suggested responses to these questions should prove helpful in planning a team-building program. For additional detailed guidance, the series of articles by Mahoney is recommended.[11–15]

Implement team building

A number of specific skills are required in effective team building. These include interpersonal skills that stress means by which groups can develop long-term relationships; skills that focus on building cooperation and mutual support; skills in substituting group goals for those of the individual; problem-solving and decision-making skills that stress group efforts; communication skills; and finally, skills in developing a whole-person philosophy of work.[16]

The overall effectiveness of any organization depends to a great extent on the healthy growth of its members. Teamwork is meaningless unless it begins with individual ability and responsibility. Although it is necessary that a group work together to perform its function, the individual must not be lost in applying the team development concept. Individual motivation is the starting point of all human productivity. Teamwork is not the goal. Teamwork is merely a means of harnessing the individual effort and contribution of persons who make up the team.[17]

Myrtle and Robertson suggest that team building be implemented by enhancing and supporting peer leadership since this accounts for well over one-half of the norm variance regarding employee range of satisfaction. They also suggest enhancing the working climate by demonstrating concern, providing autonomy and encouraging participation in decision making where possible.

In addition, they advocate exercising a leadership role that is characterized by sharing power, involving employees in discussions affecting them and promoting positive intergroup and intragroup interaction, rather than by traditional direct authority and control strategies. Finally, they believe that an effective supervisor should develop and facilitate group processes that promote shared goals, enhance mutual respect, ensure shared tasks and require ongoing development of mutual support and group cohesiveness.[18]

Evaluate and change the process

The final step in achieving group process effectiveness through team building involves periodic evaluation of progress in achieving team-building goals and initiation of changes in the team-building process as necessary. The most effective method of evaluation is to compare actual progress to planned progress.

Progress in team building will not always proceed according to plans and the supervisor's wishes. There

---

Progress in team building will not always proceed according to plans and the supervisor's wishes.

---

may be difficulties. There will be periods of collaboration and progress followed by setbacks. The supervisor's approach must be to accept the uncontrollable and control the controllable. Effective planning and appropriate attention to the details of the team-building process will minimize relapses in carrying out the program.

WORK CONTENT STEPS IN TEAM BUILDING

The two sets of steps identified in Figure 1 are separated for discussion purposes only. In practice, the supervisor and the work group would pursue the work content and the group process steps concurrently, with the objective being to improve both through systematic team-building efforts.

Because the work content steps are well known and widely used by health care supervisors, they are not

addressed in detail. For those desiring a more thorough review of the work content process, many texts are available on the management-by-objectives approach illustrated in Figure 1.[19,20]

The first step regarding the content of the work to be performed by the group is to determine the overall purpose and long-range goals of the department, section or program. This should be accomplished in accordance with organizational guidelines and should be addressed as a group process in which group members participate in determining the purpose and goals of the department.

As illustrated in Figure 1, the next step is to establish annual objectives that are derived from and support the goals. Action plans that pinpoint responsibilities and tasks in support of the objectives are then formulated. Finally, an agreed upon group structure for accomplishing the objectives is developed.

To track progress toward achieving goals and objectives, monitoring of group performance is essential. This is achieved by establishing performance measures, standards in relation to these measures and milestones by which progress can be measured over time. For example, the objective might be to reduce an error rate by 20 percent for the year, and a reduction of 5 percent might be an appropriate milestone to achieve in the first quarter of the year.

The final two steps in improving work content outcomes are periodic evaluation of the group's accomplish-

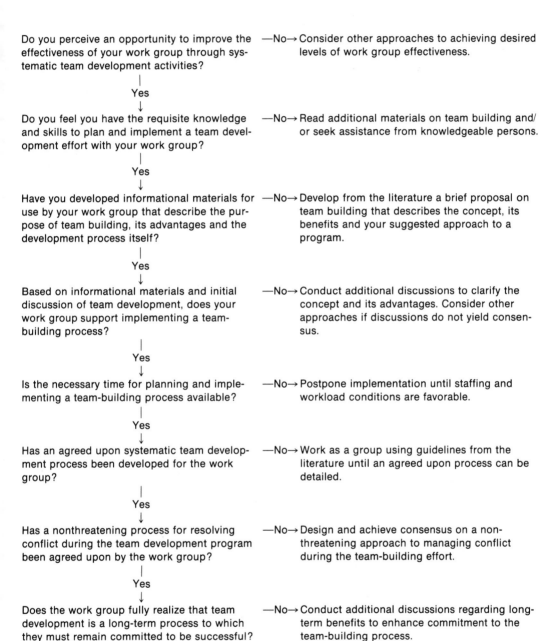

Do you perceive an opportunity to improve the —No→ Consider other approaches to achieving desired
effectiveness of your work group through sys-   levels of work group effectiveness.
tematic team development activities?

|
Yes
↓

Do you feel you have the requisite knowledge —No→ Read additional materials on team building and/
and skills to plan and implement a team devel-   or seek assistance from knowledgeable persons.
opment effort with your work group?

|
Yes
↓

Have you developed informational materials for —No→ Develop from the literature a brief proposal on
use by your work group that describe the pur-   team building that describes the concept, its
pose of team building, its advantages and the   benefits and your suggested approach to a
development process itself?   program.

|
Yes
↓

Based on informational materials and initial —No→ Conduct additional discussions to clarify the
discussion of team development, does your   concept and its advantages. Consider other
work group support implementing a team-   approaches if discussions do not yield consen-
building process?   sus.

|
Yes
↓

Is the necessary time for planning and imple- —No→ Postpone implementation until staffing and
menting a team-building process available?   workload conditions are favorable.

|
Yes
↓

Has an agreed upon systematic team develop- —No→ Work as a group using guidelines from the
ment process been developed for the work   literature until an agreed upon process can be
group?   detailed.

|
Yes
↓

Has a nonthreatening process for resolving —No→ Design and achieve consensus on a non-
conflict during the team development program   threatening approach to managing conflict
been agreed upon by the work group?   during the team-building effort.

|
Yes
↓

Does the work group fully realize that team —No→ Conduct additional discussions regarding long-
development is a long-term process to which   term benefits to enhance commitment to the
they must remain committed to be successful?   team-building process.

|
Yes
↓

Figure 2. Team development flow chart (process steps).

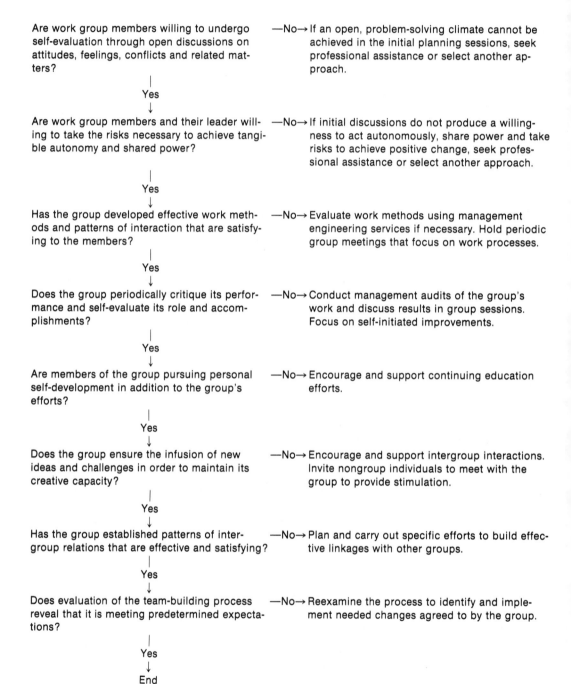

Are work group members willing to undergo self-evaluation through open discussions on attitudes, feelings, conflicts and related matters?

—No→ If an open, problem-solving climate cannot be achieved in the initial planning sessions, seek professional assistance or select another approach.

|
Yes
↓

Are work group members and their leader willing to take the risks necessary to achieve tangible autonomy and shared power?

—No→ If initial discussions do not produce a willingness to act autonomously, share power and take risks to achieve positive change, seek professional assistance or select another approach.

|
Yes
↓

Has the group developed effective work methods and patterns of interaction that are satisfying to the members?

—No→ Evaluate work methods using management engineering services if necessary. Hold periodic group meetings that focus on work processes.

|
Yes
↓

Does the group periodically critique its performance and self-evaluate its role and accomplishments?

—No→ Conduct management audits of the group's work and discuss results in group sessions. Focus on self-initiated improvements.

|
Yes
↓

Are members of the group pursuing personal self-development in addition to the group's efforts?

—No→ Encourage and support continuing education efforts.

|
Yes
↓

Does the group ensure the infusion of new ideas and challenges in order to maintain its creative capacity?

—No→ Encourage and support intergroup interactions. Invite nongroup individuals to meet with the group to provide stimulation.

|
Yes
↓

Has the group established patterns of intergroup relations that are effective and satisfying?

—No→ Plan and carry out specific efforts to build effective linkages with other groups.

|
Yes
↓

Does evaluation of the team-building process reveal that it is meeting predetermined expectations?

—No→ Reexamine the process to identify and implement needed changes agreed to by the group.

|
Yes
↓
End

Figure 2 (*continued*)

ments in relation to its work objectives and implementation of controls or changes as necessary to ensure progress toward accomplishing goals. To assist in pursuing the steps relating to improving the group's work content, a flow chart is presented as Figure 3.

This completes the group process and work content steps of team building as illustrated in Figure 1. In essence, simultaneous attention to the work content of the group and the process by which the group accomplishes its work should yield a productive, satisfied work team that

Is there agreement within the work group as to —No→ Draft, discuss and redraft the mission statement, its purpose, duties and responsibilities?   duties and general responsibilities until consensus is achieved.

|
Yes
↓

Are there clearly established goals, work objec- —No→ Establish performance objectives, measures for tives, performance measurement parameters   determining performance and standards for and standards for determining the success of   evaluating actual performance against target the work group?   goals. (A modified management by objectives program is suggested.)

|
Yes
↓

Are periodic reviews conducted to pinpoint   —No→ Establish and use milestones to measure prog- group progress and discuss issues and prob-   ress toward goals and objectives as indicators lems that may exist?   of progress or possible problems. Hold regular review meetings.

|
Yes
↓

Is the work group meeting or exceeding perfor- —No→ Develop new operating practices that enhance mance standards for productivity and quality?   teamwork. (Consider changes in staffing patterns, work flow and support systems.)

|
Yes
↓

Is the group capable of identifying and resolving—No→ Develop effective group problem-raising and most of its operational problems relating to   problem-solving techniques. (Read the literature productivity and quality?   on group problem-solving processes.)

|
Yes
↓

Are adequate controls in existence to ensure   —No→ Implement process controls and/or policies to achievement of plans that support predeter-   ensure minimum variance from plans. mined goals and objectives?

|
Yes
↓
End

Figure 3. Team development flow chart (content steps).

achieves expected successful outcomes.

SYSTEMATIC INVOLVEMENT

The overall effectiveness of a health care organization is greatly influenced by the quality of collaboration among its departmental groups and among the individual members within these groups. The extent of creative and productive contribution of such work groups to the hospital varies widely. Attaining high levels of productivity and quality while maintaining a satisfactory quality of work life presents a never-ending challenge to the health care supervisor. Few work group teams, however, are likely to develop to a level of full effectiveness without considerable nurturing and conscious development. Team development requires a planned, systematic effort by the supervisor.

In team building, the supervisor is establishing a working environment that encourages, supports and rewards voluntary involvement of personnel in the process of setting and achieving departmental performance goals and in resolving problems associated with goal attainment. Such involvement cannot be left to chance. Team building must incorporate a conscious, well-defined group effort. This involvement by personnel must be channeled such that the group can examine its own behaviors and develop courses of action to improve task accomplishment.

The objective of the team-building efforts of a work group is a results-oriented teamwork approach to the department's or section's mission. A people-oriented, open and problem-solving climate is an essential element of this teamwork. In fact, a work climate in which activities are focused more on group activity than on individual performance is the foundation upon which effective teamwork is built. Coaches of group sports such as basketball and football have long recognized this.

One can build a people-oriented, problem-solving climate and thus a more effective department by encouraging subordinates to agree upon and pursue the model process described herein as a goal toward which the supervisor and subordinates are mutually committed. Progress will be enhanced if the supervisor:

1. maintains open, two-way communication;
2. develops and continues to reinforce a spirit of cooperation;
3. seeks a contribution from each subordinate that causes him or her to be challenged but not overwhelmed; and
4. seeks and achieves mutual commitment to the objectives of the department or section and to the teamwork model as a way of effectively achieving those objectives.

Team building is a method for tapping creativity and potential and thus ensuring a greater contribution to the overall organization. Effective supervisors surround themselves with good employees and share their powers with the work group by involving members in the decisions of the department. Based on empirical research with work groups in organizations, behavioral scientists have clearly established that meaningful involvement of personnel in the decisions affecting the work group often leads to higher levels of personal satisfaction, commitment to the organization, productivity and quality.

REFERENCES

1. Myrtle, R.C., and Robertson, J.P. "Developing Work Group Satisfaction: The Influence of Teams, Team Work and the Team Approach." *Long-Term Care and Health Services Administration Quarterly* 3:2 (1979): 149.
2. Shonk, J.H. *Working in Team.* New York: AMA-COM, 1982, p. 1.
3. Baker, H.K., and Holmberg, S.R. "Stepping Up to Supervision: Building an Effective Work Group." *Supervisory Management* 27 (February 1982): 23–24.
4. Fiedler, F.D. *Leader Attitudes and Group Effectiveness.* Westport, Conn.: Greenwood Press, 1981.
5. Herzberg, F. "Productivity Begins with the Individual." *Industry Week* 211 (November 30, 1981): 84.
6. Walton, M., and Smith, G. "A Hat-Trick of Model Teams." *Health and Social Service Journal* 89 (November 9, 1979): 1453-55.
7. Herzberg, F. "Group Dynamics at the Roundtable." *Industry Week* 211 (November 16, 1981): 39.
8. Francis, D., and Young, D. *Improving Work Groups.* San Diego: University Associates, 1979, p. 6.
9. Shonk, *Working in Team*, 6.
10. Francis and Young, *Improving Work Groups*, 60–61.
11. Mahoney, F.X. "Team Development, Part 1: What Is TD? Why Use It? " *Personnel* 58 (September–October 1981): 13–24.
12. Mahoney, F.X. "Team Development, Part 2: How to Select the Appropriate TD Approach." *Personnel* 36 (November–December 1981): 21–38.
13. Mahoney, F.X. "Team Development, Part 3: Communication Meetings." *Personnel* 37 (January–February 1982): 49–58.
14. Mahoney, F.X. "Team Development, Part 4: Work Meetings." *Personnel* 37 (March–April 1982): 45–55.
15. Mahoney, F.X. "Team Development, Part 5: Procedure Meetings." *Personnel* 37 (May–June 1982): 30–41.
16. Anderson, R., and Anderson, K. "HRD in Z Type Companies." *Training and Development Journal* 36 (March 1982): 14–23.
17. Herzberg, "Group Dynamics at the Roundtable," 40.
18. Myrtle and Robertson, "Developing Work Group Satisfaction," 162–63.
19. Degan, A.X., and O'Donovan, T.R. *Management by Objectives for Hospitals.* Rockville, Md.: Aspen Systems, 1982.
20. Carroll, S.J., and Tosi, H.L. *Management by Objectives: Applications and Research.* New York: Macmillan, 1973.

Employee health services: a mutually beneficial program for facility and staff

Charlotte Eliopoulos
Vice President for Nursing
Levindale Hebrew Geriatric Center
*   and Hospital*
Baltimore, Maryland

WHEN ASKED WHERE it ranks among their issues of concern, many health care supervisors would probably place employee health low on their priority lists. After all, they must be concerned with important considerations such as service delivery, cost-effectiveness, quality assurance and resource allocation. An employee health program may be viewed as a costly luxury that can be done without. But can it? How often are supervisors faced with employees who:

- attempt to work when ill?
- injure themselves on the job?
- become exposed to communicable diseases?
- appear to be under the influence of drugs or alcohol?
- use excessive sick time?
- are restricted in their ability to perform their job responsibilities due to injury or illness?
- deny an apparent change in their health status?

Health Care Superv, 1984,3(1),37–47
© 1984 Aspen Publishers, Inc.

- display a pattern of workers' compensation cases?
- seem to be malingering?
- have sudden changes in attitude, personality or performance?
- face serious personal or family problems?

A significant amount of supervisory time and energy can be spent in managing these problems, and inappropriate management of them can result in serious risks to the employee, clients and employing agency. Thus employee health issues are more central to a supervisor's activities than may be realized.

Not only are employee health issues relevant to the supervisor's concerns, but they also significantly affect the health care industry in general. Next to heavy construction, the hospital industry reports the highest rates of illness and injury. The average employee misses several work days each year due to illness. According to the National Safety Council, there will be 6.42 injuries per 100 full-time employees with an average of 12.7 days lost per case.[1] Of every 100 employees, 3.9 will file a workers' compensation claim.[2] More than 15 percent of all employees have some personal or health problem that affects their work performance, with more than one-half of these being drug- or alcohol-related. The National Council on Alcoholism estimates that the average alcoholic costs industry anywhere from $1,500 to $4,000 annually and experiences two to three times the absenteeism of nonalcoholic employ-

ees.[3] Work-related accidents cost industry over $25 billion each year, and it is estimated that the decreased productivity and efficiency associated with employee health problems will cost another $60 billion.[4] With these realities, a strong employee health program becomes essential to any organization.

IDENTIFYING RISKS

There are a variety of health hazards in the work environment to which workers are exposed. Often these are so common that they are ignored or taken for granted. Ignorance, carelessness and thoughtlessness reduce employees' attention to protecting themselves from routine hazards and result in accidents and illness. It is important, therefore, that risks be identified and preventive measures instituted.

Infection. Because health care workers come in contact with many sick people, the likelihood of being exposed to infectious diseases is high. In addition to direct care providers who perform hands-on tasks with patients, other employees are susceptible, for example, laboratory technicians who work with specimens, laundry employees who handle soiled linen, dietary aides who carry food trays and housekeepers who must touch objects used by patients. Common infectious agents include viral hepatitis, tuberculosis, herpes simplex, Staphylococcus Aureus and enteric gram negative bacilli. Precautions such as good handwashing technique and proper disposal of wastes are important for staff to understand and practice. Employees should also be educated in the early signs of infection and encouraged to report them promptly.

Back injury. Patients are often debilitated, requiring that staff lift and transfer them. Lifting heavy objects exerts considerable force on back ligaments and can cause ligament fibers to tear; sometimes disc slippage can also result from lifting. Both types of injuries can be extremely painful and predispose the back to easier injury in the future. Good body mechanics should be taught to every new employee and should be regularly reinforced. Hydraulic lifts and other devices to ease the lifting burden are well worth the investment when compared with the decreased productivity associated with back injuries. Attention should be paid as well to other sources of back injury such as pushing food carts, throwing linen down a chute and carrying equipment or supplies.

Needle sticks. Puncture wounds from needles are the second most commonly treated injury of health care workers. Nursing employees are the most frequent group to experience needle sticks, although they are not uncommon among laundry, housekeeping and laboratory workers. An easy-to-use, conveniently located needle disposal system can aid in reducing incidents of needle sticks.

Anesthetic gases. The National Institute of Occupational Safety and Health estimates that more than 214,000 health care workers are exposed to anesthetic gases. These gases, in concentrations normally found in operating rooms, are known to reduce reaction time and sensory ability. Higher rates of spontaneous abortion and birth defects have been noted among operating room personnel, as have increased incidents of cancer, liver disease and kidney disease.[5] Gas leakage should be checked as a routine measure. Good gas administration techniques must be adhered to. Schedules to limit staff exposure time could also prove helpful.

Radiation and radioactive materials. A variety of biological effects can result from exposure to radiation, including sterility and cancer.[6] Shielding methods and monitoring of exposure are essential. (Procedural information and reports can be obtained from the National Council on Radiation Protection and Measurement, P.O. Box 30175, Washington, DC 20014.)

Ozone. This sweet-smelling gas is a chemical form of oxygen that may be generated for sterilizing rooms; some old copying machines and switchboards may also produce this gas. In addition to irritating the respiratory tract, ozone is associated with cancer. Ozone use should be carefully controlled and replaced by other methods whenever possible.

Noise. Paging systems, telephones, computers, screaming patients, floor buffers and visitor traffic are among the sources of noise in the health care environment. Noise is more than a mere annoyance—it can produce physiological stress responses in workers, evidenced by increased vital signs, indigestion, irritability and other reactions. Frequent exposure to loud noises can cause permanent hearing loss. Active control of noise in the environment should be sought, including "quiet times" when paging and equipment operation are kept to a minimum. Employees subjected to loud noise should wear protective devices.

Excessive sitting. Secretaries, clerks and receptionists perform most of their tasks while seated. Long hours of sitting can contribute to backaches, varicose veins, hemorrhoids and other problems. Poor lighting and posture while sitting can cause eye strain and fatigue. Furniture and lighting that are conducive to minimal strain should be used. Also, stretching exercises and periods away from the desk should be incorporated into the daily routine.

Excessive standing. Nurses, dentists, surgeons, laboratory technicians and other health care workers who spend considerable time on their feet are predisposed to varicosities and associated problems. Rest periods, support stockings and elimination of barriers to good circulation (e.g., garters, girdles) should be encouraged.

Heat. Laundry and dietary employees in particular may be exposed to hot work environments, which can affect cardiopulmonary function. Temperature control through the use of fans, air conditioners and equipment insulation should be instituted. Em-

ployees exposed to excessive temperatures should also be given frequent breaks.

Skin irritation. Frequent hand washing and contact with medications, detergents and other irritating substances can lead to dermatitis and nail infections. Employees should be encouraged to promptly wash irritants from skin and to use gloves when practical. Nonirritating soaps and lotions can help to reduce the amount of oil lost through frequent hand washing.

Electric shocks. Any electrically powered item, from diagnostic equipment to hospital beds to radios, is capable of producing a shock. The maintenance department should approve any electric appliance or equipment used and keep it in good repair. Regular safety rounds should be performed to detect improperly grounded equipment, overtaxed outlets and other hazards.

Wet floors. The need for a clean environment promotes frequent floor cleaning in health facilities, but wet, slippery floors promote falls. In addition, accidental spills and incontinent patients add to the risk of slips. Staff should be advised to clean spills promptly and clearly indicate wet floors.

Stress. Be it the critical condition of their patients, the amount of responsibility they hold, the monotony of their jobs or the physical effort they must exert, employees are affected by job-related stress. Stress can increase blood pressure, respiration, heart rate, blood clotting, allergic reactions, digestive problems and susceptibility to illness. Many emotional problems can also result from stress. Adequate time off, counseling, control over one's activities, opportunities for success and challenge in one's job, and maintenance of good health are among the ways stress can be reduced.

The foregoing is hardly an exhaustive list of the risks that health care employees face in their daily work; however, it should serve to demonstrate that it is not only coal miners and construction workers who are exposed to occupational hazards. The risks to health care workers are many and omnipresent. It is for this reason that a good employee health program is needed in every agency.

WHAT IS AN EMPLOYEE HEALTH PROGRAM?

Basically, an employee health program is a multifaceted, organized approach to preventing and managing health problems. In dissecting this definition the essential factors for the program are found to be:

Multifaceted. Preserving health and managing illness and injury in the work environment requires a variety of actions, including regular monitoring, investigation of incidents and illnesses, provision of education, counseling, maintaining a safe environment, sensible scheduling and realistic assignments.

Prevention. Planned and aggressive measures to preserve health and well-being are essential.

Problem management. Services should be available to assist employees with a wide range of physical, emotional and social problems.

Every agency should design an employee health program to address the unique characteristics and needs of its employee population; however, every program should include a number of standard components as outlined in the boxed insert.

One of the first steps in establishing an employee health program may be to demonstrate the importance of the program to the agency. Often administrators view the provision of anything beyond basic mandated employee health services as a costly and unnecessary luxury. Granted the program will create an additional cost, but this may be partially or even completely offset by savings in lost time, turnover, compensation claims and insurance premiums. It may be beneficial to collect all existing data on the agency's incident and accident his-

It may be beneficial to collect all existing data on the agency's incident and accident history to emphasize what health-related problems are already costing the agency.

tory to emphasize what health-related problems are already costing the agency. A hypothesis can then be drawn as to the cost benefit and cost-effectiveness of the program. (These data will also prove useful later when

Basic Components of an Employee Health Program

Preemployment examination
  Health history
  Tuberculin skin test (chest X-ray if positive or symptomatic)
  Complete blood count (CBC) with differential
  Urinalysis
  Examination for potential limitations in ability to perform job (e.g., lifting restrictions, poor vision)
Job-related injury or illness
  First aid
  Primary care or referral to appropriate provider
  Determination of ability to work after injury or illness
Health education
  Health maintenance
  Infection prevention
  Disease recognition and management
Information and referral
  Work-related problems
  Personal and family health
  Resources
Environmental safety
  Safe disposal of wastes
  Control of anesthetic gases and radiation
  Equipment checks
  Inspection for potential hazards
Surveillance
  Investigation of infections
  Review of incidents and accidents
Optional
  Immunizations
  Treatment of non-job-related illness or injury
  Annual check ups
  Special clinics or groups (weight reduction, smoking cessation, stress management, hypertension control)

The agency's specific employee health problems and needs must be determined. This can be done by reviewing incident and accident reports, excuses given for sick call-ins and insurance claims. Employees can be surveyed for their perspective on employee health problems and desired services.

Once a proposal for the specific type of program desired is obtained, the necessary resources can be estimated (e.g., an employee health service that provides primary care will require different support than one that performs only preemployment screening.) Usually, one RN per 500 employees, with physician back-up and clerical assistance, is a rule of thumb, although the services offered and availability of community resources (e.g., nearest clinic and emergency room) may indicate a different staffing pattern. The least costly level of staff to perform the program's activities should be used; for instance, a nurse practitioner or physician's assistant should be used to complete a routine physical rather than a physician; clerical staff should perform record-keeping functions and so on. The employee health service may be a division of the personnel department since it serves all departments, or in smaller agencies, may fit within the nursing department. Again, the agency needs and resources will dictate the site where services will be provided: a 16-employee agency may be able to conduct employee health activities from the nursing director's office whereas a 1,600-employee

evaluating the program's impact.) An early philosophical and administrative commitment is crucial to the development of the program.

agency may have a wing of a building as its employee health center. Provisions should be made for a reception and record-keeping area, interview office and examination and treatment room.

Written policies should be developed to guide the handling of all potential employee health problems. These policies should address issues such as

- preemployment health evaluation
- management of positive findings from examination
- tuberculosis surveillance
- management of PPD converters
- exposure to tuberculosis
- exposure to hepatitis
- exposure to other communicable diseases
- infectious employees
- management of employee with signs of infection
- management of accidents on the job
- management of illness on the job
- handling of wastes
- monitoring of radiation exposure
- immunization
- medical leave of absence
- clearance to return to work after illness or injury.

Policies must be specific, realistic and accessible to all staff. It must be remembered that the supervisor faced with an employee health problem at 2 AM needs clear policies so that appropriate action can be taken.

Good record keeping is crucial. An employee health file should exist for every employee, indicating status of the preemployment examination, results of tuberculosis tests, job-associated accidents and illnesses, and other relevant information pertaining to health status. The actions taken for positive findings should be fully documented; for example, if a suspicious spot were detected on an X-ray, a note should be made indicating that the employee was informed and chose to have it explored through a private physician. (This can also provide legal protection if the employee charges at a later date that the agency neglected to inform him or her of a positive finding and prevented the opportunity for timely treatment.) A "tickler system" on index cards can prove useful in reminding when annual screening is due and in following up problems, such as extended illnesses, infections and injuries. Of course, records of incidents, accidents, infections, sick-time utilization and safety rounds are important to maintain and analyze.

The employing agency need not be the sole provider of employee health services. Specific services can be contracted from other agencies; for example, a hospital primary care center may contract to perform entry physical examinations for a local nursing home. Heart associations, cancer societies, health departments and similar groups may be willing to provide special screening and health education programs within the agency. Group leaders may be hired or recruited from staff to conduct weight control, stress management, exercise, and smoking cessation courses. Minimal effort can mobilize considerable community resources.

LEGAL REALITIES

Employee health is more than a peripheral concern to agencies. Employers can be liable for problems caused by employees who lack adequate health to provide safe care or by physically or mentally ill employees who were insufficiently screened for employment. Employers can be liable for hazards in the work environment that predispose employees to illness or injury and for their management of ill and injured employees. Given these very real liabilities, supervisors must understand how to ensure legal protection for themselves and their agencies. Some of the more common issues that can lead to legal headaches if mismanaged are discussed below.

Preemployment screening. An employer can perform any type of reasonable health screening. Reasonable implies that the screening has a relationship to the job the employee will be performing. For example, it would be appropriate to evaluate employees' ability to lift a 15-pound box if the employees will be lifting that type of weight in the performance of their jobs; but it would not be reasonable to put a secretary or switchboard operator through that same evaluation. All employees in the same job category must also receive the same type of health screening.

Information about an individual's previous health problems must be used with care. A job applicant's history of psychiatric hospitalization, drug abuse, handicaps, injuries and other health problems may not be used as a case for not hiring if there is no residual or active problem from these conditions that could interfere with job performance. Similarly, an employer cannot ask a female about her plans to become pregnant. A careless interviewer who treads in these areas may invite a lawsuit against the agency.

The employer has a responsibility to inform employees of problems detected during the preemployment health evaluation (and during screening done thereafter). If a positive finding is present, the individual has the right to know so that treatment can be sought. Not doing so may cause the agency performing the evaluation to be charged with negligence.

Routine examinations. Basically, the same principles apply to routine screening as to preemployment screening. The examination must be related to job activities and all persons in the same job category must receive the same screening.

Evaluation of fitness to work. Employers do have the right to evaluate an employee's ability to fulfill job requirements if there is reasonable cause to doubt the employee's capabilities. For example, an employer can ask an orderly who has just returned to work after recovering from a whiplash injury to be evaluated for his ability to lift and experience unrestricted movement.

Substance abuse. The knowledge that an employee abuses drugs or alcohol is in itself not grounds for discipline or termination. Rather, how this substance abuse affects job performance and agency policy is the issue. All agencies should have policies clearly stating that employees must not use or be under the influence of drugs or alcohol while at the work setting. Employers have the right to request employees suspected of being under the influence of a substance to be evaluated (e.g., by blood sample). Of course, employers always maintain the right to send employees off duty if they are unfit for work, regardless of the cause; therefore, employees who are staggering or speaking inappropriately or who display other unusual behaviors and who deny substance abuse or refuse to submit to an examination may still be rightly asked to leave, due to questionable fitness for duty. Supervisors must be careful not to charge the employee with being drugged or intoxicated based on behavior alone. Inappropriate behavior while on duty is ample reason to refuse to allow an employee to work and can prevent a later claim that a false accusation of substance abuse was made.

Employers are obligated to recognize alcoholism and drug abuse as illnesses. Employees with these problems should be referred for help. It may be useful for agencies to develop a formal program to address the needs of these employees.

Mental illness. Like substance abuse, knowledge that an employee has a mental illness or is under psychiatric care is in itself not grounds for action. However, all employees must be able to perform their jobs correctly and behave appropriately at work, and the employee who is unable to do so has no business being in the work setting. Employees suspected or known to have emotional problems should be referred for assistance.

Pregnancy. The Equal Employment Opportunity Commission (EEOC) clearly holds that employers who fail to hire or promote, or who terminate or force leave on a woman because she is pregnant are in violation of Title VII. Morning sickness or other pregnancy-related illness is considered a legitimate reason for using sick time and cannot be denied to the pregnant woman if sick leave is an agency benefit to all employees. Pregnancy is viewed by EEOC as a temporary disability, meaning that, like other disabilities, leave of absence for this condition is not grounds for discrimination or disciplinary action. Employers cannot mandate maternity leave, e.g., stating that a pregnant woman must take leave in her seventh month of pregnancy and not return until her infant is three months old. Employers do have the right to request medical certification of the pregnant woman's fitness to work if there is concern that she is unable to perform her job. Special considerations need not be provided to the pregnant worker that would not be provided to all workers, such as extra rest periods. Also, employers cannot discriminate against a woman because she is pregnant and unmarried.

Handicaps. Agencies receiving federal funds (e.g., via Medicaid, Medicare or Hill-Burton) are required to comply with Sections 503 and 504 of the Rehabilitation Act. Basically, this regulation prohibits discrimination based on a handicap. Employers cannot subject a handicapped person to examinations or interview questions from which non-handicapped persons are excluded.

The regulation also states that employers must make "reasonable accommodations" for handicapped workers, such as altered work schedules and environmental modifications. (How far an employer must go in making these accommodations is not clear in the regulations.)

Employers are justified in not hiring or promoting or in terminating a handicapped worker for issues related to job performance. For example, a handicapped employee who has excessive absenteeism due to the handicap may be disciplined for the absenteeism providing all employees are disciplined similarly for absenteeism.

Worker's compensation. Each state has its own system for administering workers' compensation; however, there is a basic principle that is universal: all workers injured on the job,

regardless of their responsibility in causing the injury, should be compensated. All medical and hospital expenses related to the injury are the employer's responsibility. For the employee's and employer's protection, all incidents and accidents should be reported and documented. Injured employees should be urged to obtain medical attention, and if an employee refuses or states that medical care will be sought from another source, this should be documented. Never should a supervisor refuse to allow an injured employee to seek medical attention, even if that supervisor feels certain that there is no real injury.

It would be wise for agencies to review their specific state's occupational safety and health regulations with supervisory staff regularly to ensure that no unintentional violation of the law occurs.

Employee health should be an integral concern of all health care supervisors. Ensuring employee health is a major component of risk management and can prove a cost-effective strategy for an agency. Also, efforts to promote and maintain employee health demonstrate commitment and caring to employees that can yield many other benefits. A health care agency must come to appreciate that its employees are among the population it serves.

REFERENCES

1. Rabinowitz, M. "Developing and Managing a Successful Employee Health Program." In *Hospital Employee Health. Practical Solutions to Current and Potential Problems.* Atlanta, Ga.: American Health Consultants, 1982, p. 407.

2. Murray, S. "Employee Assistance Programs:

Why They Make Sense and What They Cover."
In *Hospital Employee Health. Practical Solutions to Current and Potential Problems*. Atlanta, Ga.: American Health Consultants, 1982, p. 427.

3. Zink, M. "Alcoholism: The Disease That Drains Hospital Resources Away." *Hospital Financial Management* 32, no. 11 (1978): 8, 45.

4. Murray, S. "Employee Assistance Programs," p. 428.

5. Oppman, C. "Practical Controls for Anesthetic Gases." In *Hospital Employee Health. Practical Solutions to Current and Potential Problems*. Atlanta, Ga.: American Health Consultants, 1982, pp. 134–35.

6. Coleman, K. "Radiation: New Sources/Accidental Exposures." In *Hospital Employee Health. Practical Solutions to Current and Potential Problems*. Atlanta, Ga.: American Health Consultants, 1982, pp. 231–36.

Part IV
Major Redirections

Challenging change

Jon Tris Lahti
Assistant Professor of Nursing
Division of Nursing
Mount Senario College
Ladysmith, Wisconsin

"THE implications for the nursing staff were not considered when this change was proposed." This statement summarizes the failure of an administrative effort directed toward a staffing change. The affected nursing staff was not included in planning the change. The outcome was not an improvement in nursing practice, but rather frustration and anger by those who provided the care. A few nurses actively supported the change. Others complained but offered no opposition. The remaining staff caught administration totally unprepared by strongly resisting the change—and winning.

No one should have been surprised. Changes are often well intended and perceived as good, but in the case described, the mere worthiness of the change did not prevent opposition. In fact, as Marriner notes, "Even logical, needed changes produce resistance."[1]

Health Care Superv, 1987, 5(3), 55–60
© 1987 Aspen Publishers, Inc.

Those who fought administration took a gamble. Individuals are often without legitimate power, or they perceive themselves as powerless to counter change.[2] Furthermore, any decision to oppose change is risky and can lead to loss of employment, poor performance evaluations, ridicule by colleagues, and other problems. In this case, resistance was further complicated by the fact that nurses are not perceived as being risk takers; thus, the resistance was probably unexpected.

Much of the literature offers little assistance in understanding reaction to change. Articles and texts use terms like "passive–aggressive behavior," "dangerous," and "uncooperative" to describe resisters and usually include tactics that change agents can employ to eradicate unloyal opposition. Resisters are thus viewed as those who oppose needed progress and are disruptive, antisocial, maladjusted, or worse. Lancaster and Lancaster note these perspectives as counterproductive:

Certainly not all resistance is bad; it may in fact be a warning to assess the idea carefully before implementing it further. In truth, it is usually wise to listen carefully to dissenters; their hesitancy to participate may save the change agent and organization the embarrassment of embarking on an impossible or poorly thought out strategy.[3]

To accept the notion that resistance can be beneficial, one must consider how benefit can be derived. What can potential resisters do to prevent impossible, unnecessary, and possibly disastrous outcomes that someone else is promoting?

RESISTING—AND WINNING

The key to effective resistance is planning. The following steps, although brief, provide a guideline for opposing change and winning.

Determine the rationale for change

Some reason exists for change. Usually a problem is perceived and someone has determined that its resolution requires alteration of the status quo. Resisters need to investigate two facets of the rationale. First, someone has made a comparison of what is (or is not) happening with what is supposed to be (or not supposed to be) happening. Second, someone has determined that the discrepancy is significant enough to be labeled a "problem" and, therefore, in need of resolution.

For example, suppose hospital policy requires all RNs to be currently certified in cardiopulmonary resuscitation (CPR), but only 80 percent are actually meeting the standard. As a result, mandatory CPR recertification every six months for all RNs is proposed in order to maintain the standard.

Resisters to the proposal will first determine if a problem exists. If intensive care units and emergency departments have less than 100 percent of their RNs holding current certification, then the answer is probably yes. But what if the statistic includes nursing administrators who are never involved in client care? In this case, the second facet becomes evident. Is resolution necessary when CPR skills are not required for all jobs?

In countering the proposed change, resisters must have complete information revealing both a discrepancy and a need for change. What is the organization's philosophy and mission, and is the proposed change congruent with these? How are policies being interpreted and by whom? What statistics were used? What incidents have occurred because the standard is not being met?

After an investigation, the 80 percent certification rate may be found to be out of compliance with policy but not a problem with respect to safe patient care. The mandatory recertification for all RNs, therefore, may not be necessary.

Another approach is to determine if the policies are appropriate. If not, revisions to policy can be made—a less arduous change. For example, if a revised policy states that "80 percent of all RNs will be currently certified," the discrepancy (and therefore the problem) no longer exists. Resisters might also suggest that the policy specify precisely where the 100 percent standard should be implemented, such as in intensive care, with 80 percent on other care units.

Successful resistance at this point in the change process can be beneficial with respect to allocation of resources. Further planning is unnecessary, thus saving considerable time and effort in the long term.

Review organizational constraints and resources

Successful change agents assess forces that enhance and impede change.[4] For example, clients are at less risk of fatal heart attacks if all RNs are proficient in CPR—a strong argument in favor of the change. Conversely, resources may be inadequate; budget and time may be insufficient to achieve biannual recertification.

Because of personal interest in achieving particular goals, change agents might emphasize driving forces, which facilitate the change process, while ignoring or not adequately assessing constraints that inhibit change. In addition, change agents may be goal oriented and expect that any worthy goal automatically warrants procuring all necessary resources.

Resisters must also assess driving and constraining forces and the degree to which these affect the change. Rather than merely reacting with "We don't have . . . ," resisters need to document the specific resource insufficiency. For example, 100 percent certification may be impossible given the organization's existing staff and limited budget. As a result, changes directed toward laudable but unrealistic goals are destined to fail.

Resisters can suggest goals based on the assets of the organization. For example, perhaps 90 percent, but not 100 percent, certification could be achieved given current resources. Although not congruent with policy, the change can be successful—a much sweeter taste to savor.

Analyze options

Any change includes deliberation of a number of options. Change agents identify a set of possible choices and carefully assess each. They then select the best one. But best is relative. No change is without fault, and any option can be condemned for its weaknesses. A key to successful resistance is carefully assessing the pros and cons of the same options, suggesting other options, and indicating that a better choice exists.

No change is without fault, and any option can be condemned for its weaknesses.

Resisters lose credibility when opposing change without recommending other options. This requires more than noting that the change agent's choice will never work. The point is to clearly substantiate why some other choice, including maintaining the status quo, is preferred.

Plan implementation of the option

The best option goes for naught without implementation. If resistance has been unsuccessful to this point, e.g., the boss says that "100 percent *will* be certified on a biannual basis," opposition can then fo-

cus on the implementation planning process.

Even the most detailed planning does not prevent unpredictable results. When implementation results in undesired outcomes, resisters may be tempted to cry, "I told you so." Effective resisters, however, refrain from unconstructive criticism and are prepared to offer other and more appropriate plans.

Ideally, resisters can identify those aspects of the plan that are impossible to implement or inadequate to achieve desired outcomes. From that point the plans can be thoroughly examined to ascertain the weaknesses.

For example, suppose ten additional instructors need to be hired for biannual certification. Those opposing the change conduct a market survey and determine that no more than three instructors are available. The resisters can document that unless the hospital is willing to provide costly incentives (in excess of the projected budget) to attract new personnel, the change cannot occur. Resisters can therefore recommend a delay—possibly permanent—until market conditions change.

One final approach remains: rebellion. Even in light of ethical considerations, adamant resisters may view rebellion as a last resort to frustrate change. For example, rather than attend a mandatory CPR class, staff members "discover" urgent tasks at work, become "sick" and stay home, or intentionally fail recertification testing. However, if resisters achieve success with this approach, they may earn a reputation of being unprofessional and unreliable, thereby adversely affecting their careers.

Evaluate

Although the evaluation step may seem an unlikely opportunity for successful resistance, that is not the case. Successful resisters seek to deny the change in all aspects of the process, and evaluation may provide data that indicate that the problem is not being resolved.

Change agents will consider the evaluation process, i.e., procedures for monitoring the implementation of plans, assessing change outcomes, and making any needed revisions. However, change agents do not have a monopoly on evaluation methodology.

Resisters should make sure that the evaluation mechanisms are fully developed and implemented. If resisters believe that the evaluation process is inadequate, they should suggest alterations or develop their own tools to be used jointly with other procedures.

Implicit in evaluation is accurate and timely feedback. Resisters must ensure that change agents receive only pertinent, accurate information and be constantly alert for rumors and false statements that may impede resistance efforts. In addition, resisters can request project updates, seek formal representation on committees responsible for evaluation, and hold their own meetings to maximize the potential for input and remain abreast of current progress.

WHEN ALL ELSE FAILS . . .

Implicit in these recommendations is the need for resisters to work within the system—actively collaborate with change agents—toward mutually agreeable outcomes. However, does resistance end when it fails to achieve its purposes? The answer lies in assessing benefits against costs.

When all else fails, resisters must reflect on the costs of continued opposition before decisions regarding activities outside the system are initiated.

When all else fails, resisters must reflect on the costs of continued opposition before decisions regarding activities outside the system are initiated. For example, suppose the biannual recertification policy is implemented in spite of well-organized opposition. Someone proposes a "sick-out" to bring the issue to the public's attention, hoping that forces external to the organization will demand repeal of the policy.

The protest may be successful; however, the long-term ramifications cannot be ignored. When moving beyond the boundaries of organizational policies and norms in extreme actions such as strikes or going public, resisters may be regarded with disdain by administration, colleagues, and patients. Credibility can be lost, adversarial relationships promoted and future opportunities for effective resistance diminished.

Resisters do not need to indulge in extreme actions or even achieve a clear victory to be able to claim success. A single battle may be lost, but the war can be won by creating an environment in which those who promote change must appreciate the significant positive benefits that resistance offers.

•   •   •

Resistance is critically necessary to the promotion of effective change, and those who choose to take the risks of challenging change can be valuable assets to an organization. However, effective resistance is predicated on knowledge of the change process and skill in mounting a rational challenge. Only through careful consideration of each step of the process will resisters find their efforts rewarded.

REFERENCES

1. Marriner, A. *Guide to Nursing Management.* St. Louis: Mosby, 1984, p. 82.
2. Brooten, D., Hayman, L., and Naylor, M. *Leadership for Change: A Guide to the Frustrated Nurse.* Philadelphia: Lippincott, 1978, p. 56.
3. Lancaster, J., and Lancaster, W. The Nurse as a Change Agent. St. Louis: Mosby, 1982, p. 20.
4. Lewin, K. *Field Theory in Social Science.* New York: Harper & Row, 1951.

The impact of mergers on employees

Carole A. Fink
Vice President of Nursing Services
Quakertown Community Hospital
Quakertown, Pennsylvania

A LL MERGERS ARE potentially traumatic to a considerable degree. Some mergers, however, turn out to be more traumatic than others because of the way certain key considerations are—or are not—addressed. Many published articles have addressed the financial impact of mergers, but only a few have given full consideration to the human resource aspects of mergers. Because mergers are a relatively new phenomenon in health care but have been occurring in the public sector for many years, it should be possible for health care organizations to learn from the successes and failures of mergers in business.

MERGERS IN PRIVATE BUSINESS AND IN THE HEALTH CARE SECTOR

Private business

A merger occurs when two or more organizations combine their assets to form a new entity. An acquisition results when one

Health Care Superv, 1988, 7(1), 59–67
© 1988 Aspen Publishers, Inc.

entity buys out or otherwise absorbs another.

Corporate mergers and acquisitions are occurring more frequently today than at any other time in the history of commerce. During the last decade, 23,000 mergers and acquisitions were consummated, with a total value of approximately $398 billion. Eighty-two of the acquired firms were Fortune 500 companies.[1] The ten largest mergers in 1984 directly affected the lives of more than 250,000 employees.[2] By 1990, in the financial industry alone, 3,400 banks and savings and loan associations will be involved in mergers affecting the lives of another 822,000 people.[3]

Mergers occur for several reasons. The most common reason is financial, that is, to take advantage of economies of scale and improve the "bottom line" or net profit.

Regardless of the reason for the merger, two frequent results of mergers are restructuring and downsizing. An August 4, 1986, *Business Week* cover story stated the announced cutbacks among 15 Fortune 500 companies accounted for a total of 128,000 lost jobs.[4] Additional cutbacks, many due to mergers, are now announced on a regular basis. Although eliminating jobs is an old story for U.S. companies, the new story is the growing willingness of some of the most successful corporations to slash management and professional jobs.[5]

In addition to downsizing, pyramids are toppling as companies eliminate layers of management in hopes of becoming leaner and meaner.[6] Major reorganization and restructuring is being undertaken to increase productivity.

The health care sector

During the past five years, major changes in Medicare reimbursement have forced hospitals and other health care providers to look at cost containment as never before. Consumer demands for greater efficiency and an increased competition for the health care dollar are but two of many factors that are making mergers in the health care sector more popular. Health care experts have predicted that by 1995, out of the 5,800 currently existing community hospitals, 1,023, or 18%, will close for financial reasons.[7] Mergers are enabling some hospitals to become more financially profitable and are helping others to simply survive.

Two other predictions relating to merger activities in hospitals are that (1) the industry will be downsized by 17.6% over the next ten years as a result of a decline in inpatient utilization and (2) there will be 479,000 fewer hospital full-time equivalents.[8] Obviously, mergers in health care will have a tremendous human resource impact just as they have had in private business.

Approximately 20.7% of all hospitals in the Northeast have already merged. In the Southwest, 29.8% of all hospitals have merged. Many other hospitals throughout the United States are currently investigating the feasibility of mergers.

LIABILITIES TO ORGANIZATIONS FACING MERGERS

Major employee concerns

How will all this merger activity affect employees? Three elements act as liabilities to organizations facing mergers.[9] First, workers view mergers as a major life change that negatively affects their behavior. Second, the increase of unproductive behavior demands the most refined and strategic sorts of inter- and intraorganizational communications. Many organizations have faulty communication systems, even under the best of circumstances. Third, during a merger there exists an increased need for perceptive human resource planning.

For most people, merger planning is a period of uncertainty and insecurity.

When companies merge, the advantage looks good, especially for the major stockholders. The disadvantage, the impact on employees, is frequently overlooked in the excitement of change. This is unfortunate, because to a large extent it is the employees who ultimately determine whether mergers work.[10,11]

Mergers and the rumors associated with them lead to a number of concerns for the employee. The major concern is how the merger will affect them in both the short and long term.[12] For most people, merger planning is a period of uncertainty and insecurity. Lower-level employees and executives alike wonder how the merger will affect their jobs. Emotions generated by the uncertainty and insecurity can result in altered behavior, decreased morale, reduced productivity, stress, illness, accidents, conflict on and off the job, and a total lack of commitment to making the merger work.[13]

Several major factors contribute to the employee's response to mergers.

Mergers mean change

Resistance to change seems to appear most often in the following situations: electronic and technological changes, procedural changes, reorganization, environ-mental changes, and rapid corporate growth or decline.[14] Mergers involve some, and sometimes all, of these changes. In addition, mergers frequently bring many, and often unanticipated, changes in management.

Eight of the factors that provoke resistance include the following:[15-17]

1. *Loss of control.* As individuals, we want to be in control of our lives. Each person's need for security is different. A change that may seem insignificant to one person may precipitate a strong negative response in another. This loss of control could lead to feelings of powerlessness and meaningless-ness and eventually lead to varying degrees of alienation.[18]

2. *Social losses.* When informal relationships among employees are threatened because of an organizational change, employee resistance to the proposed change results.

3. *Loss of status or esteem.* Some of the more subtle status symbols may not be recognized by others, for example, a "minor" change in title from Director to Assistant Director (with no change in responsibilities) after reorganization or a relocation of a desk, positioning it farther from administrative offices.

4. *Economic loss.* Sometimes a change has present or future monetary implications for an employee—loss of jobs or "flattened" organizations with fewer job opportunities for promotion.

5. *History of stability.* In some instances, a company's history of stability may work against it when it comes to implementing change.

6. *Inconvenience.* The need to learn and adjust to a new procedure is an inconvenience that often prompts resistance from employees.

7. *"Surprise" factor.* Resistance is often the first response to something totally new and unexpected that employees have had no time to prepare for mentally.
8. *A real threat.* Sometimes the threat posed by the change is a real one.

Resistance to change may be minimized or even eliminated by following these six guidelines:

1. *Provide advance notice.* Make sure employees understand the reason for the change and any benefits to the organization and themselves. Any potential disadvantage should also be discussed.
2. *Phase in changes slowly.* Give employees the opportunity to get adjusted to the change.
3. *Consider friendships and status.* Protect both whenever possible. Try to view the situation from the other person's perspective.
4. *Encourage employee participation.* Whenever possible, and especially if resistance is expected, invite affected employees to assist in making the decisions necessary to implement the change.
5. *Provide an opportunity for discussion.* Sometimes a change is clearly for the worse. Providing an opportunity for employees, either individually or in groups, to air their feelings will minimize nonproductive activity and griping.
6. *Be open to new ideas.* Serve as a role model if you expect others to be flexible and adapt readily to change.[19]

Mergers create stress for the individual

To date, neither researchers nor managers have systematically addressed and examined merger stress and its consequences.[20] A merger creates a number of potential and powerful antecedents of stress—stressors.

Whether these stressors create stress and its resulting negative outcomes depends on the characteristics, predisposition, and goals of the employees involved as well as the organization's plan for systematically intervening and helping employees manage merger stress.[21,22]

Merger stress can have a number of negative consequences for both the individual and the organization. Physiologic responses to a merger may include fatigue, over- or undereating, use of drugs or excessive intake of alcohol, high blood pressure, migraine headaches, muscle aches, sleeplessness, trembling, or muscle tics. From an emotional perspective, one typical merger stress response is preoccupation. Depression, anxiety, chronic indecisiveness, vague feelings of helplessness, malaise, or loneliness may also occur.[23,24]

To help the employee cope with job stress, encourage the employee to do the following:

- Build resistance through regular sleep, exercise, and good health habits.
- Compartmentalize work and nonwork life. Develop noncareer competencies.
- Work hard on the job, but when at home learn to blank out job problems.
- Talk through problems on the job with peers. If necessary, seek professional help.
- Withdraw physically from the situation for a while; take a break.
- Learn and practice relaxation techniques.[25,26]

Successful executives often rely on the following seven characteristics or abilities, described as "qualities of success" to offset job stress. These characteristics could apply to some extent to all employees within the organization.[27]

- *Recognition and practice of frustration*

tolerance. "All that work and nothing to show for it" is a statement that often precedes rage and frustration. The successful person is able to work hard on a project knowing that all the hard work might lead to nothing in the end.

- *Encouragement of participation.* Pressure can be shared by encouraging others to participate in the control and development of a project.
- *Self-questioning.* Persons who hold themselves in high esteem try to understand their mistakes without becoming upset over their personal responsibility for them.
- *Living with your competition.* When competing with colleagues for specific objectives, there is no reason to become hostile toward those individuals. It is a part of the game. It is necessary to learn to handle hostility.
- *Mastery of victory and defeat.* Victory is not a reason for excessive celebration. Nor is defeat a reason to feel that this is the end of one's career.
- *Identification with groups.* Part of the strength required to withstand pressure derives from a person's relationship to coworkers and supervisors as a group.
- *Realistic goal setting.* One's level of aspiration must be in line with capabilities and the realities of a situation. It may be necessary to examine career choice during this period.

Mergers may change existing culture

There are five elements that make up a strong organizational culture: business environment, values, heroes, rites and rituals, and cultural network.[28] Although a merger may affect any or all of these elements, concentration on a merger's effect on

the values of the organization is in order because the existing values of a hospital are readily and seriously threatened by a proposed merger.

Values are the basic concepts and beliefs of an organization that form the heart of the corporate culture.[29] The power of values lies in the fact that people care about them. This power can pose a problem as well as serve as a source of strength.[30] Three risks assumed when building or reinforcing the shared values of an organization's employees include the following:

1. *The risk of obsolescence.* One of the most serious risks of a strong system of shared values is that economic circumstances may change while shared values continue to guide behavior in ways no longer helpful to the organization's success.
2. *The risk of resistance to change.* A company with a powerful growth mentality may have problems in a cost-containment climate.
3. *The risk of inconsistency.* To build a strong culture, top management must be convinced that it can adhere faithfully and visibly to the values it intends to promote.

A nationwide survey of American managers found that shared values related to the following:

- *Feelings of personal success.* Managers who reported greater compatibility between their personal values and the values of the organization reported experiencing significantly greater feelings of success in their lives.
- *Organizational commitment.* Managers who felt that their values were particularly compatible with those of the organization were significantly more confident that they would remain

with their current employer for the next five years.

- *Self-confidence in understanding personal and organizational values.* As managers' perceptions of a close alignment of personal and organizational values increased, so did the extent of their awareness and understanding of the organization's values.
- *Ethical behavior.* As value compatibility increased, so did the extent to which respondents agreed that their organizations were guided by highly ethical standards.
- *Feelings of job and personal stress.* Managers in the low shared values category reported higher levels of job-related anxiety spilling over into their personal (home) lives.
- *Organizational goals.* In general, the goals of an organization were seen as more important by those who felt their values were aligned with the organization than by those who felt that their values were not consistent with their organization's values.[31,32]

If it is necessary to change the culture, the following five strategies may help:

1. Recognize that peer group consensus will be the major influence on acceptance of change or willingness to change. One of the strongest influences on people is the influence of their personal ties with others.
2. Convey and emphasize two-way trust in all matters related to change (especially communications). Communications are better in high-trust situations. Because of this, change initiated by an insider often takes place much more quickly than change urged by an outsider.
3. Think of change as skill building and concentrate on training as part of the change process. Even if people understand and accept a change, they often do not have the required skills and abilities to carry out the new plan.
4. Allow enough time for the change to take hold. It may take ten years for a megacorporation to change its culture.
5. Encourage people to adapt the basic idea for the change so that it will fit the real world around them. Employees need to be able to be "out of control" comfortably.[33]

There are also several levers human resource managers can pull to gain a values advantage in their organization. The most useful of these are programs to clarify and communicate values, recruitment and selection of the right employees to fit the organization and relevant orientation for those employees, proper training in the proper skills, reward systems that tap intrinsic motivation, and counseling support, especially if the new values in the culture are different from those formerly held by the employee.[34]

Mergers may contribute to organizational burnout

Organizational burnout can occur when an organization's leaders burn out, its nonsupervisory employees burn out, or when neither leaders nor employees burn out, but when a system or circuit failure occurs—usually related to ineffective communication or the lack of clearly defined organizational goals accepted by the employees.[35]

Signs and symptoms of organizational burnout include bickering, a sense of resignation, stagnation, lack of vision, incompetency (which can result in dysfunction, "witch hunting," or a tremendous amount of time and energy spent on appearances rather than results), a low level of mutual trust, frustration, lack of follow-up and back-up, inefficient use of resources, poor communication, fear, and an unwillingness to take reasonable risks.

Besides the lack of interest and the institutional inertia that may exist, more serious

---

Early strategic planning can prevent organizational burnout following a merger.

---

consequences can emerge in the form of aggressively overt actions against the organization by an alienated or disgruntled group.[36]

Mergers foster the type of burnout caused by system failure. Some major problem areas are the organizational chart, that is, one that fails to clarify lines of responsibility or communications; unclear or inadequate organizational controls; the lack of a system for financial awards and incentives; and overall inadequate communication.

Early strategic planning can prevent organizational burnout following a merger in the following ways:

- *Participation.* Strategic planning can provide an opportunity and forum for different groups and management levels in the organization to express their views and be involved in the planning.
- *Identity and direction.* The strategic planning process forces the organization to engage in a critical analysis of itself. The willingness of an organization to subject itself to constructive self-criticism to a large extent determines how successful it can be. Organizational burnout many times is caused by an organization's self-delusion,

very often a perception of itself as something more grandiose than it may actually be.

- *Proaction rather than reaction.* If the strategic planning process is conducted properly, an organization can anticipate many of the adverse conditions it is likely to face in the future and can thus examine various options to overcome them before projects are actually implemented.
- *Discipline.* Often, organizations invest sizable sums of money and other resources in a new activity but fail to devote appropriate time, effort, or resources to examining the results. Strategic planning can provide an effective mechanism for a timely objective review of the projects implemented.
- *Objectivity.* With participation, strategic planning provides an opportunity for the organization to examine complex and sensitive issues (and suggested projects) from a more objective basis.
- *Innovation and creativity.* Strategic planning helps organizations to think about issues in an organized and systematic manner. It should include not only an economic analysis of the merger and its effect, but also supporting analyses based on administrative and personnel concerns.[37,38]

Additional strategies to minimize impact of mergers on employees

Activities and programs that address the emotional needs of the employee during and following a merger should be the responsibility of all organizations involved in the merger. Twelve recommended general strategies are

1. *Timing.* If legally possible, announcement of the merger proposal's approval so that employees of all organizations involved hear it internally before the news media break the story.
2. *Meetings.* Encourage all managers to meet frequently and regularly with their staffs throughout the transition, even if they have no concrete information about the merger to share at every meeting. Communication makes the most important contributions to the success of a merger. Honest, frequent communication (oral and written) enhances a feeling of security and helps reduce rumors.
3. *Anonymous feedback.* Establish a telephone merger hot line, preferably staffed by the personnel or training department, so that employees can call anonymously to express concerns and ask questions.
4. *Manager training.* Conduct a seminar or miniseminar for managers on how to help employees and themselves cope with the changes and uncertainty of the transition period. The training program might include general topics such as the nature of change, creating rational perceptions, coping with loss of control, and how to retain good employees.
5. *Technical job training.* Anyone whose job will change as a result of the merger should be trained as early as possible before consummation of the merger.
6. *Family assistance program.* Establish an employee and family counseling program (perhaps through a local mental health agency) and subsidize it.
7. *Stress reduction.* Conduct or sponsor seminars on how to recognize and deal with stress.
8. *Counterparts.* As soon as employees feel comfortable with the idea, arrange introductory social meetings in which counterparts from the merging organizations can meet and get acquainted. This helps eliminate the "we versus they" attitude.
9. *Orientation.* When legally permissible, conduct orientation programs about the merging organizations. Information will reduce fear of the unknown.
10. *Explanation of new roles.* As opportunities and options for employees are identified, make them known immediately. People's primary concern is whether they will have jobs.
11. *Help for those who will lose their jobs.* Provide outplacement services for displaced employees. Help them deal with the trauma of impending unemployment.
12. *Postmerger team building.* Begin team building efforts as soon as the merger is complete. Team building needs to take place from top to bottom in the new organization.[39,40]

•   •   •

Few people are likely to escape involvement in some aspect of a merger sometime during their careers. In both private business and health care, communication is a critical factor. The role of the first-line manager is especially crucial because of the manager's proximity to the employees "in the field" and "on the floor." Managers who are sensitive to the needs and feelings of their employees during a merger can help to literally make or break the merger.

REFERENCES

1. Schweiger, D.L., and Ivancevich, J. "Human Resources: The Forgotten Factor in Mergers and Acquisitions." *Personnel Administrator* (November 1985): 47–61.
2. Ibid.
3. Dull, J., "Helping Employees Cope with Merger Trauma." *Training* 23 (January 1986): 71–73.
4. Nussbaum, B. "The End of Corporate Loyalty?" *Business Week* (August 4, 1986): 42–49.
5. Ibid.
6. Zemke, R. "Delayed Effects of Corporate Downsizing" *Training* 23 (November 1986): 67–68, 73–74.
7. Cherskov, M.M. "What's Driving Upcoming Mergers." *Hospitals* (January 5, 1987): 36–40.
8. Ibid.
9. Sinetar, M. "Mergers, Morale, and Productivity." *Personnel Journal* (November 1981): 863–67.
10. Dull, "Helping Employees Cope with Merger Trauma."
11. Schweiger, and Ivancevich, "Human Resources: The Forgotten Factor in Mergers and Acquisitions."
12. Ibid.
13. Dull, "Helping Employees Cope with Merger Trauma."
14. Oramer, D.S. "Winning Employee Cooperation for Change." *Supervisory Management* (December 1985): 18–24.
15. Kanter, R.M. "Managing the Human Side of Change." *Management Review* 74 (April 1985): 19–21.
16. Oramer, "Winning Employee Cooperation for Change."
17. Money, W., Gilfillan, D., and Duncan, R. "A Comparative Study of Multi-Unit Health Care Organizations." In *Multihospital Systems: Strategies for Organization and Management*, edited by M. Brown and B. McCool. Rockville, Md.: Aspen Publishers, 1980, p. 381.
18. Ibid.
19. Oramer, "Winning Employee Cooperation for Change."
20. Schweiger, and Ivancevich, "Human Resources: The Forgotten Factor in Mergers and Acquisitions."
21. Ibid.
22. LaBier, D. *Modern Madness*. Reading, Mass.: Addison-Wesley, 1986.
23. Schweiger, and Ivancevich, "Human Resources: The Forgotten Factor in Mergers and Acquisitions."
24. LaBier, "Modern Madness."
25. Simendinger, E., and Moore, T. *Organizational Burnout: Strategies for Prevention and Change*. Rockville, Md.: Aspen Publishers, 1985.
26. LaBier, "Modern Madness."
27. Simendinger, and Moore, *Organizational Burnout*.
28. Deal, T.E., and Kennedy, A.A. *Corporate Cultures*. Reading, Mass.: Addison-Wesley, 1982.
29. Ibid.
30. Ibid
31. Ibid.
32. Posner, B.Z., Kouzes, J.M., and Schmidt, W.H. "Shared Values Make a Difference: An Empirical Test of Corporate Culture." *Human Resource Management* 24 (Fall 1985): 295–301.
33. Deal, and Kennedy, "Corporate Cultures."
34. Kouzes, and Schmidt, "Shared Values Make a Difference: An Empirical Test for Corporate Culture."
35. Simendinger, and Moore, *Organizational Burnout*
36. Ibid.
37. Simendinger, and Moore, *Organizational Burnout*.
38. Money, Gilfillan, and Duncan, "A Comparative Study of Multi-Unit Health Care Organizations."
39. Dull, "Helping Employees Cope with Merger Trauma."
40. Robino, D., and DeMeuse, K. "Corporate Mergers and Acquisitions: Their Impact on HRM." *Personnel Administrator* 30 (November 1985): 33–44.

Planning and implementing a staff reduction

William Weimer
*Vice President for Personnel
    Services*
*Ohio Hospital Association
Columbus, Ohio*

Paul W. Cutlip
*Corporate Vice President for
    Human Resources*
*Marymount Hospital
Garfield Heights, Ohio*

THE ANNUAL rate of increase in hospital costs has diminished since 1982, and inpatient admissions and length of hospital stay have likewise decreased. New technology and new treatment methods are making it possible to shorten inpatient stays and are offering new choices for less costly ambulatory treatment.

One result of recent trends in hospital activity has been the reduction of the hospital work force in various parts of the country. Hospital employment has decreased both nationally and in Ohio for the first time since the mid-1940s. From the first quarter of 1983 through the fourth quarter of 1984, Ohio's hospital work force dropped by nearly 10,000 full-time-equivalent employees—a reduction of 5.8 percent of the work force.[1]

Sound, equitable staff-reduction policies are necessary in today's hospitals. Such policies should be in place before reductions occur, and

Health Care Superv, 1986,5(1),56–70
© 1986 Aspen Publishers, Inc.

they should ideally be put in place with supervisory understanding and involvement.

Establishing a clear policy with respect to the definitions of layoff and reduction in force is a primary concern. There are dangers in layoff policies; thus policy definitions must be clear. Job security is a major issue for unions, and any hospital's layoff or reduction policy must be defensible in court. The National Labor Relations Act protects anyone on "layoff" status, and anyone with a "reasonable expectation of recall" can vote in a union election.

In choosing between true layoff and reduction in force, reduction— permanent separation from the organization—is the better choice if there is little realistic chance of recalling the workers in the foreseeable future.

Most union contracts call for layoff by seniority. However, straight seniority simply does not work in the hospital situation. Skill, ability, and performance must be taken into account in any layoff or reduction procedure.

DISCRIMINATION

The Equal Employment Opportunity Act, Title VII of the Civil Rights Act, and related state laws present most of the problems associated with staff reductions. Race discrimination is a potential problem in any reduction procedure, particularly if the reduction is "direct by classification" without bumping. Subcontracting out a particular function presents the same potential discrimination problem.

Performance evaluations are usually a poor basis for a layoff policy; they are often too weak to use in defense against a discrimination charge. There are wide variations in supervisors' approaches, and evaluations are not always completed uniformly. Disciplinary and attendance records are also often too weak to use in defending against a discrimination suit.

There are many situations to avoid with respect to sex discrimination charges arising from staff reductions. Any explicit or implicit gender-related reason for removal from the work force is a clear Title VII violation. Regardless of traditional job roles, gender is rarely a bona fide occupational qualification.

Discrimination because of handicap (Section 504 of the Rehabilitation Act) is also an important consideration. The development of a reduction policy must also consider whether the procedure involves reasonable accommodation for the handicapped worker.

Age discrimination can be a severe problem with management employees, and the resulting lawsuits are often vindicative. Age-discrimination charges must be actively defended against by the employer; otherwise, the hospital is open to additional charges. Time, effort, and expense are the real problems associated with age-discrimination suits. Note, for example, that an employee who retires before age 70 may be eliminated for consideration for rehire simply because he or she has already retired.

The Employee Retirement Income Security Act (ERISA) is probably the most complicated employee-relations law on the books, and there are important ERISA implications in releasing employees who are eligible for retirement. The protection afforded by ERISA may also be triggered by an organization's severance pay plans.

It is often standard procedure when facilities or entire departments close completely to limit the reduction in force to those who are not eligible for pensions. However, if no severance pay goes to people who are vested, while others do receive such pay, there may be ERISA problems. The courts have said that such practices constitute age discrimination and have ordered severance pay for retirees.

Early retirement plans or "window plans" that offer people a limited time to exercise a special retirement option must be voluntary; otherwise, they are age discriminatory. The voluntary nature of such a plan must be provable in court.

Employment at will—the right of an employer to fire at any time for any reason, or for no stated reason at all—is a rapidly eroding concept. Related laws vary from state to state and sometimes county to county. Wrongful discharge actions carry the potential for both civil and punitive damages. Age discrimination, slander, and libel often make up a "standard" wrongful discharge suit. Thus the or-

Age discrimination, slander, and libel often make up a "standard" wrongful discharge suit.

ganization must clean up its policies and update the language in its employee handbook, particularly in areas where employment at will still applies. Even in employment-at-will areas, however, one cannot legally discharge an employee for being absent to perform a legal duty such as jury duty or testifying in court.

It is with the foregoing legal and policy pitfalls in mind that the following questions and guidelines were developed. A staff reduction is not to be entered into without thorough preparation. However, with adequate planning—meaning observance of all pertinent laws and close attention to details—a reasonable and generally equitable way can be found to accomplish this unwelcome task with the minimum possible amount of disruption and aftereffects.

DEVELOPING A LAYOFF POLICY AND PROCEDURE

I. General considerations
   A. Should efforts be made to avoid a layoff?
      1. Have all the administrative, real, and hidden costs and savings of a layoff been calculated?
      2. What are the hospital's future plans?

3. What do economic forecasts show?
4. What will the effect be on the hospital's good will and reputation, employee morale, patient care, and professional recruiting efforts?

B. If efforts to avoid a layoff are indicated, have such efforts been made?
1. Regular work time has been reduced.
   a. All or some full-time employees work fewer hours.
   b. Full-time employees are converted to part-time.
   c. Shorter workweeks are mandated.
   d. Increased vacation time is permitted.
2. Early retirement is encouraged.
3. Use of paid and unpaid time off is permitted.
4. Use of overtime is restricted.
5. Paid time off (vacation, holiday) is used without replacement of employees.
6. Hiring freezes (attrition procedure) are enacted, with reassignment of personnel.

C. Has the hospital identified and articulated the objectives of its layoff policy? The layoff policy should contain a statement of the intent, objectives, and general philosophy of the policy.
1. An effort to protect the job security of as many employees as possible has been made.
2. The highest quality of patient care has been maintained.
3. Employees who may be affected by layoff are given fair and equitable treatment.
4. Decisions are made without regard to race, creed, national origin, sex, or age.

D. How will employees be informed that they have been laid off?
1. Telephone call
2. Personal interview
3. Letter sent to last-known address by either registered letter or regular mail
4. Names posted in public place

E. Will the process vary if the particular employee is on vacation or sick leave?

F. When will layoff notice become effective?
1. When mailed
2. When received

G. Will the employees be given a specified amount of advance notice of the reason, extent, or duration of the layoff, if possible?

H. Will employees be able to

appeal the decision? If so, how? Will there be any time limitations?

I. What will be the duties of laid-off employees upon their receipt of the layoff notification?
   1. Inform management of desire to be recalled
   2. Return hospital-issued equipment and vacate office or desk
J. Have responsibilities been delegated for each step in the layoff procedure?
K. Have the departments or units to be affected been identified?
   1. Identified essential positions
   2. Identified targeted positions
L. What effect will the layoff have on fringe-benefit entitlements?
   1. Health care insurance
   2. Life insurance
   3. Long-term disability insurance
   4. Dental insurance
   5. Retirement
   6. Educational-assistance program
M. What will be the effect of the layoff on accrued but unused vacation and holiday time available at the time of layoff? What about accruals during layoff?
N. Will laid-off employees be entitled to any financial assistance?

1. Will severance pay be provided?
2. Are the laid-off employees informed that they are eligible for unemployment compensation unless they decline an offer of suitable employment for which they are qualified?
O. Will counseling or other assistance be made available to laid-off employees?
   1. Benefit options
   2. Health insurance
      a. Retain "balance-of-month" coverage employer has already paid for
      b. Become dependent upon spouses' plans
      c. Continue under existing group plan by paying entire premium
      d. Convert from group plan coverage to an individual plan
      e. Enroll in short-term insurance plans
         (1) Short-term plan—60 days to one year
         (2) Fixed-benefit hospital and surgical plan
         (3) Major medical plan
         (4) Individualized plan
   3. Unemployment compensation

a. The company will notify the local unemployment office of the employee layoffs.
b. The employee will be supplied with information regarding benefit eligibility.
c. An unemployment compensation officer will be invited to the hospital.

4. Food stamps
5. Public aid
6. Child eligibility for reduced-price school lunches
7. Free or low-cost medical care
8. Free legal aid services
9. Budgeting and credit advice
10. Mortgage terms (some banks may stretch out terms)
11. Property taxes (county assessor may have authority to grant delay)
12. Car payments (repayment plan)
13. Utility payments (deferred payment or assistance)
14. Life insurance policies (use of dividends and cash value to pay premiums on personal whole life policies)
15. Reduce food budgets (food banks)

16. Credit cards
17. Reduce transportation costs (reduce automobile insurance, use car pools, sell extra car)
18. Outplacement efforts
    a. Send letters of recommendation
    b. Send letters confirming layoff
    c. Contact potential employers or employment agencies

P. Have the employees been informed of any obligations they will have during the time they are laid off?
1. Notice of a change in address, telephone number
2. Notice that they no longer wish to be considered for recall
3. Notice of any illness, accident, relocation, or new job that would prevent recall

Q. Have all the legal ramifications of the layoff policy been considered?
1. Antidiscrimination laws
2. Unemployment compensation
3. Safety regulations
4. Labor agreements
5. Other federal and state laws
6. Other guidance by legal counsel

R. Will there be communication with the community or press?

II. Layoff considerations
  A. What method will be used to determine which employees will be laid off?
    1. Length of service (seniority)
    2. Employment status (temporary, casual, probationary, part-time, full-time)
    3. Performance
    4. Skill or ability
    5. Management discretion
    6. Combination of the above
  B. Will different methods be used for different departments or job classifications? Will exceptions to a hospitalwide policy and procedure be made for particular departments or job classifications (e.g., employees with special skills)?
  C. If length of service is to be used to determine individual layoffs, has "length of service" been adequately defined?
    1. When does length of service begin?
    2. When does it terminate?
    3. How will part-time seniority be determined— by date of hire or by hours worked?
  D. If length of service (seniority) is to be used to determine individual layoffs, which level of seniority, e.g., hospitalwide, department, or job classification, will be used in determining the order of layoff?
  E. If length of service is to be used, what happens if two or more employees have the identical length of service?
    1. Use of other considerations
    2. Management discretion
    3. Lottery
  F. If employment status is used to determine individual layoffs, will provisions be made for layoff by seniority within levels, e.g., temporary employees first, then probationary employees, then standby employees, then regular part-time employees, and lastly regular full-time employees?
  G. If performance is to be used to determine individual layoffs, can the hospital validly measure such? Do the hospital and the work force have confidence and respect in the currently used performance appraisal system?
  H. If skill and ability are used to determine individual layoffs, how will skill and ability be defined?
    1. Licensure
    2. Training
    3. Previous experience
    4. Management discretion
  I. Should the layoff policy contain a statement that employees who remain after the layoff must be able to perform the available work?

J. Will voluntary layoffs be encouraged?

III. Transfer and bumping considerations

  A. Will there be a provision in the layoff policy for laid-off employees to transfer by seniority, employment status, or performance to existing vacancies for which they are qualified, rather than being laid off?

  B. Will different departments or job classifications be subject to different bumping policies and procedures? Will certain departments or job classifications be exempt from a general hospitalwide bumping procedure?

  C. If bumping is permitted, which of the following options will be selected as the bumping procedure?

    1. Laid-off employees may bump by hospital seniority, employment status, or performance into the same or lower classification in which the employee has training or experience

    2. Only laid-off employees with a certain amount of seniority (e.g., one year) may bump, and they may only bump an employee with less hospital seniority in the same or a lower job classification

    3. Bumping is restricted to cases of permanent layoff

    4. Only the least-senior employee in a job classification can be bumped by a laid-off employee, provided the laid-off employee has greater hospital seniority

    5. A laid-off employee can bump an employee with less hospital seniority in a lower classification in the same department

  D. Will the layoff policy state that the laid-off employee has a specified period of time (e.g., five working days) to decide to exercise transfer or bumping rights before being laid off?

  E. What will be the status of the bumped employees? What rights will they have? Will they be treated as laid-off employees and have the right to bump other less senior employees?

IV. Recall procedure

  A. What will be the order of recall?

  B. Will the layoff procedure specify that recall is in reverse order of layoff by level of seniority, e.g., hospital, department, or classification or employment status, provided that the recalled employee can perform the available work?

  C. Will the layoff procedure provide that, if a vacancy occurs in a classification where no employee is on layoff, then the most senior-qualified employee on lay-off who can perform the work will be offered the position before the hospital posts the job or recruits outside?

D. If a full-time employee took a part-time position rather than being laid off, will this person have preference over laid-off employees when a full-time job for which he or she is qualified becomes available?

E. If a part-time employee took a full-time position rather than being laid off, will this person have preference over laid-off employees when a part-time job for which he or she is qualified becomes available?

F. How will the laid-off employees be notified of a recall?
1. Telephone
2. Registered letter or regular mail

G. When a laid-off employee is recalled, how much time (e.g., two weeks) is allowed for reporting to work before being considered a voluntary resignation?

H. May a laid-off employee decline a recall offer and maintain layoff status, or is this considered a voluntary resignation?

I. If a laid-off employee can decline a recall offer and

still maintain layoff status, how many times can he or she do so?

J. How will recalled employees be placed? Does the layoff policy provide that a laid-off employee will be recalled only to the same or a lower job classification and the same department and only if able to perform the duties of the job to which he or she is being recalled?

K. What are the obligations of the hospital and the employee upon recall?
1. Benefits reactivated
2. Pay rate based on new position, old position, or both
3. Employee to give notice of changed circumstances (address, telephone number, health, marital status)

L. How will an employee's recall affect seniority with respect to future layoffs? Will all or part of the time the employee was laid off be considered as part of his or her length of service?

M. What are the rights of a recalled employee vis-à-vis employees who remain laid off? If an employee is recalled into a new position and the old position then becomes available, is the person entitled to the former position before qualified, laid-off employees with less seniority?

N. How long is a laid-off employee maintained on layoff status before being terminated?

NONBARGAINING STAFF REDUCTION, REASSIGNMENT, AND RECALL POLICY

If for economic reasons it becomes necessary to implement a cutback in hospital employment, the following factors will apply in determining which employees will be affected: (1) job classification; (2) length of continuous hospital service; and (3) ability and fitness to perform the required work. An employee's ability and fitness to perform required work refers to having the basic qualifications required in the position description and being able to meet the minimum job requirements of the job after one week.

Employees affected by a staff reduction will be recalled to work in the reverse order of the reduction; that is, the last employee reduced from the staff shall be the first employee recalled. Employees having the same reduction date shall be recalled in order of length of service.

Employees affected by staff reduction who are not able to return to their job classifications shall be given an opportunity to fill vacant positions for which there is no recall list and for which they may be qualified by expe-

Employees affected by a staff reduction will be recalled to work in the reverse order of the reduction; that is, the last employee reduced from the staff shall be the first employee recalled.

rience, education, or training. This shall not supersede the hospital's promotion and transfer policy.

Staff reduction may require that employees who are not affected (laid off) be reassigned to different shifts, departments, or schedules. When this is necessary, the hospital will make every effort to protect more senior employees as related to reassignment.

I. Staff reduction, reassignment, and recall procedure
   A. Definition: the staff reduction review committee is a body comprised of the president, senior vice president, personnel director, and the appropriate administrative officer for the department or job classification affected.

II. Procedure
   A. Reduction
      1. Administrative staff, in conjunction with the manager of the department affected, shall
         a. Determine the most effective mix of job classifications or skills

necessary for reduced operation

b. Where more than one cost center is involved, determine optimal mix in each department (e.g., X-ray diagnostic, X-ray therapy, and nuclear medicine; all nursing divisions)

c. Determine the required number of hours to be reduced by job classification

d. Set reduction-effective date

e. Provide number of hours to be reduced by job classification to personnel

2. Personnel department shall review seniority listing within the job classification to determine affected individual employees.

B. Determination shall be made in the following order:

1. Hospital length-of-service order (shortest length of service first). This shall be based upon hospital seniority (last term of continuous uninterrupted service).

2. Employees with the same length of hospital seniority will be reduced by performance based on supervisor's written recommendation and past performance appraisals.

3. Employees in affected job classifications with no scheduled hours (e.g., as needed, contingency, overload pool) shall not be utilized during staff reduction unless employees on staff reduction are not available for work.

C. Department head shall

1. Notify affected employees of the last day worked; this shall be performed with the personnel representative and shall follow the staff reduction interview procedure

2. Notify employees of benefit options, available assistance, and recall policy

3. Document complete justification for retaining an employee if the affected employee is one whose loss would seriously affect the hospital's ability to complete its mission requirement as defined

4. Submit justification to staff reduction review committee

D. The staff reduction review committee shall

1. Review the request

2. Review the justification

3. Determine importance of an individual to meeting the hospital mission requirement

4. Review relevant personnel files

5. Make the final determination

6. Advise the department head of the decision
7. Document the decision

STAFF REDUCTION GUIDELINES

I. Outline of guidelines
   A. The department head will schedule a meeting with the employee and a personnel department representative.
   B. During the interview, the employee will be made aware of open positions for which he or she would qualify.
      1. If the employee applies, is selected, and takes such reassignment, that employee will have rights, by length of service, to return to his or her original position if it becomes vacant.
      2. If the gross wages of the position offered are lower than 90 percent of the gross wages of the position the employee occupies, the employee will have the right to accept or reject the position. If the position is rejected, the employee shall retain his or her place on the recall list.
      3. If the scheduled hours on the personnel requisition exceed 20 percent over or under the number of scheduled hours the affected employee had while working, the em-
ployee will have the right to accept or reject the position. If the position is rejected, the employee shall retain his or her place on the recall list.
      4. If the gross wages of the position offered are within 10 percent of the wages and hours are within 20 percent of the number of hours of the position the employee occupied, the employee may accept or reject the position. If rejecting the position, the employee will, in effect, be resigning and will waive all recall rights. There will be no extension of benefits; all benefits will be cancelled the first of the month following termination.
      5. If there are no vacant positions, the employee will be notified of last day worked and benefit options, available assistance, and recall policy.
      6. The personnel representative will make available a letter of reference to the employee.
      7. The personnel representative will offer to assist the employee in writing a resume.
      8. The personnel representative will review the hospital's recall procedure with the employee.

C. Benefits
  1. Two-week notice pay at employee's current rate of pay will be given. As possible, each employee will be offered the alternative of working an additional two weeks with pay or ceasing active work immediately and receiving the equivalent amount as notice.
  2. All benefits for remainder of month in which layoff occurs will be paid.
  3. Hospitalization insurance for one month following layoff will be paid.
  4. The employee will have the option of paying premiums for hospitalization insurance for an additional five months at hospital's group rate.
  5. Accumulated vacation and holiday pay may be paid on the day of separation.
  6. The employee shall not lose accumulated sick leave time during the period of staff reduction. However, sick leave time shall not be payable during such time.
  7. Accumulation rights
    a. The affected employee shall not accumulate benefit time during a period of staff reduction.
    b. As it applies to basic vacation eligibility, laid-off period will not reduce the accrual.

II. To minimize disruption of employee work hours consistent with operating efficiency, the following actions shall be undertaken:
  A. The department head shall
    1. Determine approximate mix of
      a. Day, evening, and night employees
      b. Full-time and part-time employees
      c. Part-time scheduled hours ratio per employee
      d. Work-unit assignment of employees
    2. Obtain employee listing by hospital length of service
    3. Determine appropriate reassignment of personnel considering:
      a. Length of hospital service
      b. Willingness of employee to adjust hours, shifts, unit, etc.
      c. Amount and extent of changes required
      d. Personnel department review of recommended changes
  B. Guidelines for reassignment
    1. Senior employees may, by hospital seniority, displace the least-senior employee in the same job classification on the same shift or unit. An effort shall be

made to find a position with the same or similar hours.

2. The least-senior employee displaced shall be assigned to the most appropriate unit, shift, or schedule as determined by the department head. Such employees shall have no displacement rights over other employees.

3. When the only positions available are substantially different than what a more senior employee is presently working (e.g., a 40-hour employee and an 8-hour weekend position), the senior employee will be offered such position or reduction status with recall rights.

C. Personnel department shall
1. Provide job classification listing by length of service to department head
2. Review recommended changes to ensure fairness and consistency

Voluntary reduction of hours policy

During periods of reduced census or workload, an employee desiring a reduction of scheduled hours may request such reduction from the immediate supervisor. Approval for such reduction shall be obtained from department administration, and notice shall be given to the personnel department in writing. There shall be no loss of benefit accrual for an employee who voluntarily reduces hours. Voluntary reduction of hours shall not exceed three months.

In the event that more employees request voluntary reduction of hours than is necessary to meet the workload reduction, hospitalwide length of service in each department shall be the determining factor. Employees with the greatest length of service shall be given priority.

Voluntary time off is not designed to excuse employees of absenteeism or tardiness or to result in questionable overtime practices.

Economic separation

When it is apparent that permanent elimination of departments, classifications, or jobs must occur, and there is no reasonable expectation that the employees affected may be placed in other positions in the hospital or be recalled to work in one year or less, permanent economic separation shall be instituted. Employees permanently separated from the hospital shall be eligible for all appropriate benefits (accrued vacation pay, holiday pay, personal days, and severance pay equal to the amount of vacation eligibility). However, such employees will have no recall rights to the same or a similar position.

An employee affected by an economic separation will, however, be placed on a priority rehire list and will be contacted by the personnel department if and when a position becomes available for which the separated employee may be eligible through experience, training, education, or other qualifications. Priority rehire consideration shall apply for a period of one year.

A. The personnel department shall
  1. Post and process the approved personnel requisition in accordance with hospital posting policy.
  2. Review the list of employees on reduction status in the same job classification after internal transfer or promotion process is complete and a requisition is to be filled from outside.
  3. Determine, in reverse order of reduction, the employees eligible for recall to the position. Note: employees with the same reduction date shall be recalled by length of service (i.e., longest service first).
  4. Determine if a current employee might be qualified for the opening if there are no employees on the recall list in the job classification on the requisition.
  5. Contact the employee to determine his or her interest if it is possible to recall a laid-off employee to same job classification.

  a. Employees shall be offered positions based on reverse order of reduction, regardless of number of scheduled hours on the requisition.
  b. If the scheduled hours on the requisition exceed 20 percent over or under the number of scheduled hours the affected employee had while working, and if the gross wages of the position are not within 10 percent of the employee's original wages, the employee will have the right to accept or reject the position. If the position is rejected, the employee shall retain his or her place on the recall list.
  c. If the scheduled hours on the personnel requisition are within 20 percent of the number of scheduled hours the employee had worked, and if the gross wages of the position offered are within 10 percent of the position the employee occupied, the employee must accept the position or lose recall rights.

REFERENCE

1. American Hospital Association. *National Panel Survey—Ohio Portion, 1981–1985.* Chicago: AHA, 1985.

Index

Notes

Notes

Notes

Notes

Notes

Notes

Notes

Notes

Notes

Notes

Notes

Notes

Notes

Notes

6563

Notes

Notes